"This is a highly readable book ... cl
McCarthy provide the latest information and present a new, inno-
vative, comprehensive, biopsychosocial approach to the treatment of
premature ejaculation, the most common male sexual disorder. I
recommend it highly."

> —Pierre Assalian, MD, director, Human Sexuality Unit,
> McGill University Health Center and president of the
> 17th World Congress of Sexology, Montreal, 2005

"This is the most comprehensive guide to dealing with premature
ejaculation I have ever seen! It addresses subtypes, cognitive, emotional, and behavioral components, medical issues, relapse, and the
ever-important influence of the couples' relationship on the cause and
cure of this disorder. Drs. McCarthy and Metz have not only done a
great service to couples experiencing this problem, but to sex therapists as well. I will definitely recommend the book to my clients and
will incorporate its exercises in my treatment protocol."

> —Jean D. Koehler, Ph.D., president, American Association
> of Sex Educators, Counselors, and Therapists (AASECT)

"*Coping with Premature Ejaculation* is chock-full of great suggestions
for improving one's sex life. Written by two experienced sex therapists, the book offers sound advice and sensible suggestions for gaining control over ejaculation and, more importantly, for becoming a
better lover!"

> —Sandra R. Leiblum, Ph.D., director, Center for Sexual
> & Relationship Health, UMDNJ-Robert Wood Johnson
> Medical School.

"Finally, an updated, comprehensive guide for a problem that affects
millions of men and their partners. These highly respected authors in
the field of sex therapy bring years of clinical experience and insight
to these pages in a format that's masterfully helpful. This is a great
book, and I plan to recommend it to all my patients who struggle with
premature ejaculation."

> —Dennis P. Sugrue, Ph.D., past president of the American
> Association of Sex Educators, Counselors, and Therapists
> (AASECT) and coauthor of *Sex Matters for Women*.

Coping with Premature Ejaculation

How to Overcome PE, Please Your Partner & Have Great Sex

MICHAEL E. METZ, PH.D.

BARRY W. McCARTHY, PH.D.

New Harbinger Publications, Inc.

Publisher's Note

This publication is designed to provide accurate and authoritative information in regard to the subject matter covered. It is sold with the understanding that the publisher is not engaged in rendering psychological, financial, legal, or other professional services. If expert assistance or counseling is needed, the services of a competent professional should be sought.

Distributed in Canada by Raincoast Books

Copyright © 2003 by Michael E. Metz and Barry W. McCarthy
New Harbinger Publications, Inc.
5674 Shattuck Avenue
Oakland, CA 94609

Cover design by Amy Shoup
Edited by Jessica Beebe
Text design by Tracy Marie Carlson

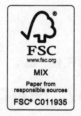

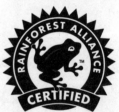

ISBN-10 1-57224-340-6
ISBN-13 978-1-57224-340-8

New Harbinger Publications' website address: www.newharbinger.com

15   14   13
20   19   18   17   16

We want to express our gratitude and deep respect for the several thousand men and couples we have clinically worked with over the years. They invited us into their private lives, opening honestly to their personal and sexual distress. While we can only thank them anonymously, they have led us to develop a more comprehensive understanding of premature ejaculation. We thank our patients who have been the "pathfinders" for this new approach. This book presents the result of what we have learned from them and from the scientific research and clinical efforts of our sex therapy colleagues. We hope we have learned well enough and that this book will be helpful to others with PE.

We also want to acknowledge the outstanding contributions of the people we have happily worked with at New Harbinger Publications: Spencer Smith, acquisitions editor; Jessica Beebe, copy editor; Amy Shoup, art director; Gretchen Gold, web manager, permissions, and advertising; Troy DuFrene, marketing and sales; Michele Waters, director of production; and Heather Mitchener, editorial director. Thank you all.

—Michael E. Metz
—Barry W. McCarthy

Contents

1

Understanding Premature Ejaculation

What is premature ejaculation (PE)? You might expect that this is an easy question to answer, but it depends on whom you ask. Masters and Johnson (1970), the founders of modern sex therapy, stated that a man has PE if he ejaculates before the woman reaches orgasm in 50 percent or more of their sexual encounters. PE is sometimes defined as a problem accomplishing a "normal" length of time between insertion and ejaculation. Studies have even defined PE by a specific amount of intercourse time: less than one minute, two, three, four, five, seven, or ten minutes, each amount based on a different reason. Still others have proposed to define PE by the number of intra-vaginal thrusts: eight thrusts, fifteen thrusts.

The best professional description of PE is that *the man does not have voluntary, conscious control, or the ability to choose in most encounters when to ejaculate.* We think this is the most helpful definition because conscious control reflects the interpersonal, cooperation, and intimacy issues for couples better than some mechanical or numerical definition.

Contemporary popular culture dictates that to enjoy sex maximally, the man should be able to last at least an hour during intercourse! Such myths about sexual performance are among the most negative influences on male and couple sexual satisfaction.

Kevin and Monica had the most common sexual problem facing young couples. Kevin suffered from PE. Both blamed Monica's non-orgasmic response on Kevin's PE. They believed that if Kevin could last longer, Monica would easily be orgasmic during intercourse. Sex would be perfect every time. It was Kevin's duty as a man to make sure Monica had an orgasm during intercourse each time—an extraordinary pressure on Kevin and his penis.

Kevin did some Internet research and read how easy it was to cure PE. All he had to do was practice the squeeze technique (which we do not recommend), in which the man or his partner squeezes the underside of the tip of the penis to delay orgasm. He was very hopeful, but that broke down within two weeks. Kevin was stymied, and Monica resented his being a technician rather than an involved lover. Sex was no longer fun; it was a chore. Kevin was frustrated with Monica and with himself. He thought that everyone else quickly developed ejaculatory control. What was wrong with him? Or was it her fault? Maybe they did not love each other and this was a doomed relationship. Would PE destroy their marital bond?

Our Comprehensive Approach

If you are facing PE in your relationship, and especially if you are a couple who has tried the common techniques for treating PE and failed, we offer you our extensive experience, our clinical knowledge, and a detailed approach to treating PE. Our approach integrates the body, mind, and relationship aspects of PE to help you appreciate the complexity of your problem, develop understanding for yourself and your partner, build empathy for each other's experience of PE, and create a detailed plan to organize your efforts to change. This biopsychosocial approach will not only help you overcome rapid ejaculation but deepen your intimacy and sexual joy.

Testing Your Knowledge of PE

How much do you really know about PE? Take this true-false quiz before reading further.

True   False   Most men engage in intercourse for twenty to thirty minutes.

True   False   A good lover prolongs intercourse until his partner has an orgasm.

True   False   Women function like men: they have a single orgasm during intercourse.

True   False   Men who ejaculate after two to seven minutes of intercourse have poor ejaculatory control.

True	False	PE is caused by too much masturbation, especially during adolescence.
True	False	Thrusting alone is enough for most women to have an orgasm during intercourse.
True	False	PE is always caused by psychological problems.
True	False	To deal with PE, the woman needs to be less erotic and the man has to reduce arousal.
True	False	PE is nature's way of increasing fertility.
True	False	PE is a symbol of a relational power struggle.

In fact, each of these items is false. Old and new myths about PE abound. In this book we will confront myths, including that PE is a simple, painless problem; intentional; purely psychological; the woman's fault; a sign of sexual inadequacy; caused by masturbating too much or too fast; a sign of hostility; a symbol of male selfishness; the same for everyone; a problem with only one cause and one treatment; and a hopeless problem.

The Truth about PE

PE is the most common male sexual problem. The majority of male adolescents and young adults begin their sexual lives as premature ejaculators. Most men, as they gain experience, do develop ejaculatory control. However, approximately three in ten adult males regularly experience PE.

The good news is that PE can be understood and changed. You can increase your sexual satisfaction—and your partner's—by learning to control ejaculation. The challenge is to deal with the complex, multicausal, multidimensional problem of PE and to enjoy sex with enhanced ejaculatory control.

Kevin and Monica were approaching PE from a poor understanding of the problem and a self-defeating focus on sexual performance. At its essence, sexuality is about sharing pleasure, not passing a performance test. Healthy, integrated sexuality values intimacy, pleasuring, and eroticism. Like most males, Kevin believed that sex was about eroticism, frequency, and proving adequacy to himself or to the woman. Kevin hadn't really thought about sex as a way to share pleasure and to build intimacy. Yet, the reality is that PE affected both Kevin and Monica.

Successful treatment combines taking individual responsibility for sexuality and being an intimate sexual team. Understanding and changing PE was primarily Kevin's responsibility; Monica did not cause Kevin's PE, nor could she change it for Kevin. She *could* help Kevin honestly and objectively assess the components of his PE and be seriously involved in the change process.

PE is not a simple problem with one cause and one solution. There are actually nine different types of PE. PE involves biological, psychological, and relational factors, both in its causes and in its effects. A successful change program must address all the relevant factors. A successful program must also include a plan for dealing with relapse. Our approach is effective because it helps you address all of these issues.

It is helpful to realize that you are not alone. Guilt, stigma, blame, and counterblame are unnecessary and will subvert your motivation to resolve PE and enjoy couple sexuality.

Understanding Male Sexuality

It was once believed that the more masculine you were, the faster you ejaculated. But there is more to sex and sexuality than your penis, intercourse, and orgasm. Sexuality is about sharing and enjoying affection, pleasuring, intimate playfulness, eroticism, intercourse, orgasm, tenderness, and passion for life.

The great advantage of male sexuality is that young males find desire, arousal, and orgasm easy and predictable. Adolescents are encouraged to value sexuality as an integral part of masculinity. Men learn sexuality as automatic and—for better or worse—autonomous. In other words, the man needs nothing from the woman to achieve desire, arousal, and orgasm.

This view of sexuality becomes problematic as the man and the relationship age. Healthy sexuality is intimate and interactive, not autonomous. Learning ejaculatory control is an interpersonal process, not an individual one.

What You'll Need to Learn

What do you need to learn about PE and ejaculatory control? First, this is a couple task. The woman plays an integral role in learning ejaculatory control. Second, ejaculatory management exercises are built on the solid foundation of nongenital and genital pleasuring. Ejaculatory control is not about the man performing up to a perfectionist standard or proving he can give the woman an orgasm during intercourse, but about developing a mutually satisfying couple style that includes pleasure-oriented intercourse. Learning ejaculatory control should not mute or decrease pleasure. To the contrary, it will expand physical pleasure as well as pleasure in the relationship.

There are several crucial skills in learning ejaculatory control.

Physiological Relaxation

The first skill is to learn how to relax your body during sexual arousal. Physiological relaxation is the foundation for your body's healthy sexual functioning.

Identifying the Point of Ejaculatory Inevitability

The second skill is to learn to identify the point of ejaculatory inevitability. After that point, orgasm is no longer voluntary. Even if your mother-in-law walks in or something happens which is a sexual turnoff, you will still ejaculate. Actually, the point of ejaculatory inevitability is the beginning of the three- to ten-second orgasmic response. Many men report the most sensations and feelings just a second or two before they ejaculate. The ability to identify the point of ejaculatory inevitability is crucial in the techniques we'll teach you.

Ejaculatory Regulation

The third skill is learning to regulate your ejaculation. We will teach you the two basic approaches: *excitement toleration* and *excitement saturation*. In excitement toleration, you will learn to maintain high levels of arousal without going on to ejaculation. With excitement saturation, you will learn to focus on your own bodily sensations, patiently welcoming the pleasure, allowing your body to become saturated or flooded with physical pleasure while slowing ejaculation by maintaining physical relaxation. You will then have reasonable control over when you ejaculate.

Cooperation for Intimacy

The fourth skill is to cooperate as a couple. Our approach to PE works best when you and your partner work together. The point of all these efforts is to enhance your closeness, comfort, pleasure, and joy as a couple.

Increasing Pleasure

The fifth skill is to enhance your pleasure, not reduce it. Do-it-yourself ejaculatory control techniques emphasize distracting yourself and reducing arousal—for example, by wearing two condoms, using a desensitizing cream on the head of the penis, thinking anti-erotic thoughts about debt or cleaning bathrooms, or using distraction techniques such as going over baseball scores or multiplication tables. These do reduce arousal but do not enhance ejaculatory control because they disconnect your awareness (the primary source of control) from your sensations and body. In addition, they carry the risk of causing a more severe sexual problem, erectile dysfunction.

Our approach to treating PE might seem counterintuitive because the exercises involve increasing penile and erotic pleasure. But you'll find that increased awareness leads to increased control. We emphasize taking in erotic sensations and feelings, not shutting them out.

Most men can benefit from training in ejaculatory control. Instead of viewing PE as a major problem that makes you inadequate or makes the woman feel that her sexual needs are ignored or neglected, think of ejaculatory control as a skill the couple—not just the man—can learn in order to enhance mutual sexual satisfaction.

Letting Go of Your Focus on Performance

In movies, sex is always perfect. Both people are highly aroused before touching even begins; sex is flawless, nonverbal, and intense; they quickly have simultaneous orgasms and continue to make love all day. Our discussion about PE is scientifically accurate, sex-positive, helpful, and relevant to real couples, but it will not be made into a movie or sell as a romantic story. We are not describing a perfect fantasy model but what really goes on in a healthy sexual relationship. By its very nature, couple sexuality is variable. If the only purpose of sex were orgasm, men and women would masturbate and not engage in a relationship or intercourse. Masturbation is easier, more predictable, and more in your control than couple sexuality. Yet the great majority of men and women prefer couple sex to masturbation.

Giving up the performance-focused approach frees you to learn ejaculatory control and enjoy couple sex. Having a reasonable amount of control over when you ejaculate and enjoying the orgasmic experience is very different than making sure your partner is orgasmic during intercourse before you are allowed to have an orgasm. Since one in three women who are regularly orgasmic are never orgasmic during intercourse (Foley, Kope, and Sugrue 2002), this expectation is obviously flawed. Just as important, when you are so obsessed with performance, you cannot enjoy sharing the pleasure of intercourse. Rather than enjoying orgasm, you are judging your performance.

Your focus on performance can become a major distraction for your partner. While she may be distracted from pleasure by her own unreasonable expectations, such perfectionist sexual goals interfere with your positive feelings about sex and about each other, and ignore the reality of variable sexual response. You are not a perfectly functioning sexual machine. You are a sexual man with changing and complex thoughts, behaviors, and feelings. You are not a rock or an island. You are involved in an interpersonal sexual relationship. Remember, the ultimate goal of learning ejaculatory control is increased sexual and relationship satisfaction. In understanding the role of sexuality in a relationship, desire and satisfaction are more important than arousal and orgasm.

The Myth of One Cause, One Treatment, and Easy Cure

The pop psychology belief about PE is that it has one cause (masturbating too much and too fast and approaching couple sex the same way), that there is one treatment (the squeeze technique), and that change is quick and easy. Recently, a simplistic medical approach has appeared which assumes that treating the man with antidepressant medication alone will retard ejaculation. This requires no learning by the man and no participation by the woman.

Human sexual behavior, including PE, is multicausal and multidimensional, with large individual and couple differences. The best way to understand PE is as a physical, cognitive (mental), behavioral, emotional, and relational phenomenon that can involve a number of causes and interactive effects. It is crucial to address all the factors which contribute to your type of PE so that you can approach the problem successfully and avoid slipping into old feelings, thoughts, and behaviors about PE.

It is risky to use a medication or a do-it-yourself technique like a penile desensitizing cream and not involve your partner or even tell her what you are doing. Even if this approach works and you don't ejaculate as quickly, if you stop taking the medication or using the cream, PE will likely return and might even be worse. What does that do to your partner and relationship? She may blame you and be angry, feeling you could delay ejaculation, but now you just don't want to. She may view you as selfish and not caring about her sexual feelings. If you're not approaching the problem as a team, a relapse can leave you both demoralized and trapped in a blame-counterblame pattern.

Relational Issues and PE

Relational problems can be a cause of PE, a result of PE, or both. Even when PE is caused by a medical problem or a physical injury, the frustration and sexual stress affects your relationship. Ideally, the man would learn and share information about PE with his partner. Unfortunately, that is the exception rather than the norm. Ideally, the woman would be empathic and supportive and be an active ally in trying to understand and resolve PE. Unfortunately, the woman may be unsure and alternate between blaming herself and blaming her partner. She might react in an extreme way, becoming overly sympathetic and "motherly," which is antierotic, or becoming angry and demanding, which is intimidating and increases performance anxiety.

In learning ejaculatory control, most couples benefit from working to increase communication, understanding, empathy, cooperation, and intimacy. This reinforces the concept that sex is more than genitals, intercourse, and orgasm. Sexuality accounts for 15 to 20 percent of overall relationship satisfaction. Sexuality should not be a deal maker or deal breaker for the relationship, as there are other crucial facets to love and intimacy. Sexuality can enhance your relationship and make it special. PE works against that process.

Improving ejaculatory control is worthwhile for you and your relationship. The core of a relationship is a respectful, trusting, cooperative friendship enriched by emotional and sexual intimacy.

What if you do not have a partner, or have a tenuous relationship in which you and your partner can't work together to learn ejaculatory control? Our approach can still offer helpful information, guidelines, and understanding. In addition, you can use the self-exploration and masturbation exercises to learn and practice the skills of physiological relaxation, identifying the point of ejaculatory inevitability, and maintaining awareness at high levels of arousal.

When you're seeking a new relationship, it's important to choose a partner you are attracted to, comfortable with, and trust would be an ally in learning ejaculatory control. Many men with PE are so embarrassed that they avoid a sexual relationship, settling for one-night stands and either ignoring the problem or apologizing for their sexual performance. You need to approach the woman as a "sexual friend." Disclose the problem without apologizing. Tell her that her sexual feelings and needs do matter to you, and request that she be a cooperative, sharing partner in working together to improve ejaculatory control and make this an enjoyable sexual relationship. Your leadership is essential in the process of change.

Understanding Female Sexuality

The major sexual complaint of men—that the woman is not orgasmic during intercourse—is not a sexual dysfunction but a normal variation of female sexuality. Female sexual response is more variable and complex than male sexual response. This does not mean better or worse. The man usually has one orgasm which occurs during intercourse. The woman might be singly orgasmic, nonorgasmic, or multiorgasmic, and orgasm might occur during the pleasuring or foreplay phase, during intercourse, or through afterplay.

Rather than expecting that the woman respond like him—have one orgasm during intercourse without needing additional erotic stimulation—the man needs to understand and accept that only one in four women respond in that manner (Foley, Kope, and Sugrue 2001). Orgasmic response is a healthy, integral part of female sexuality, but orgasmic response patterns are variable. Few women are orgasmic 100 percent of the time. For women, sexual satisfaction includes orgasm but is less rigidly tied to it. The majority of women find it easier to be orgasmic with manual, oral, rubbing, or vibrator stimulation than through intercourse. In fact, the most common sexual response pattern is for the woman to be orgasmic with manual or oral stimulation during the pleasuring phase, with the man being orgasmic during intercourse.

To develop the intimate team approach that will help you overcome PE effectively, you will need to understand, accept, and affirm your partner's patterns of arousal and orgasm. She has to develop her "sexual voice," not in reaction to what you think is right, but as a way to express her feelings and preferences. Together, you create a sexual relationship which is equitable and respectful of individual preferences rather than based on a simplistic view of male-female sexual differences.

Men grow up with the idea that they are supposed to be the sexual experts and it is their job to be sure the woman is sexually satisfied. We encourage you to consider a very different way to be in an intimate relationship. Your partner is the expert on her sexuality. Her desire, arousal, and orgasm are her responsibility, not yours.

The old definition of a good lover was a man who took responsibility for the woman's sexual satisfaction and was able to last long enough so that he could give her an orgasm through intercourse alone. The healthier, more realistic definition of a good lover is the man who accepts the woman as an equal sexual person and intimate partner.

As a good lover, you are open to her sexual requests and guidance. Each person's sexual enthusiasm and arousal feeds the other's desire, arousal, orgasm, and satisfaction. The man enjoys intercourse for himself and the relationship. He is aware and involved in giving and receiving pleasure during intercourse. Intercourse can involve a range of positions and movements that add to the intimate, interactive process. Being orgasmic is a natural extension of the arousal process. Sex does not end with his ejaculation. There is an afterplay phase in which he is open to her feelings and requests.

The man who is learning ejaculatory control with the goal of ensuring that the woman has an orgasm during intercourse is setting himself and the relationship up for failure and frustration. The reason to improve ejaculatory control is to make the sexual experience more pleasurable and satisfying for both partners, not to prove something to yourself or your partner. If she is orgasmic during intercourse and that is her preference, enjoy it. However, it is poison for you, the woman, and the relationship to put pressure on yourself to last longer so you can give her an orgasm during intercourse. The focus of ejaculatory control is to enhance the entire sexual experience: awareness, comfort, intimacy, pleasure, eroticism, intercourse, orgasm, and afterplay.

PE and Other Sexual Problems

Although it might feel overwhelming to tackle more than one sexual problem, PE often involves other sexual problems too, and you'll be more successful in dealing with PE if you consider these problems along with PE.

Coexisting Sexual Problems in Men

For men, the most common coexisting sexual problems are *acquired inhibited sexual desire* and *acquired erectile dysfunction. Acquired* means that the man once experienced desire and erections, but now they are problematic or nonexistent. Couple sex therapy is the treatment of choice for both of these problems. Many men would rather first try to resolve the problem using this book's guidelines and exercises. If that is not helpful within three to six months, then agree to consult a sex therapist.

Acquired Inhibited Sexual Desire

The key to sexual desire is positive anticipation and feeling you deserve good sex for you and your relationship. The usual reason for male inhibited sexual desire is frustration and embarrassment over a sexual dysfunction, especially erectile problems. Occasionally, inhibited desire may be caused by medical illness or side effects of medications, disappointment with the partner or relationship, alcohol or drug abuse, depression or anxiety, relationship stress or alienation, lack of couple time or energy, and preoccupation with children, extended family, or career. You'll need to identify the factors that inhibit your sexual desire and actively confront and change them.

Many men feel so badly about PE that they fall into the cycle of anticipatory anxiety, tense and unsatisfying sex, and sexual avoidance. Sexual desire cannot be treated with benign neglect. Avoidance just feeds the negative cycle. The hormone which most influences sexual desire, *testosterone*, works on a feedback system. Sexual activity enhances testosterone, while stress and sexual avoidance decrease testosterone.

In rebuilding male sexual desire, the key is to reinforce the cycle of positive anticipation, pleasure-oriented sexual experiences, and a regular rhythm of sexual encounters. You subvert your own sexual desire when you view sexual intercourse as a pass-fail test or tell yourself that anything less than a perfect sexual performance means you are less of a man. Desire is about connecting with your partner and sharing sexual pleasure.

Acquired Erectile Dysfunction

Erection problems are a major cause of male inhibited sexual desire. The traditional view of male sexuality is that a real man is able to have sex with any woman, any time, in any situation. This unrealistic demand is self-defeating for the man and his penis. In fact, by age forty, 90 percent of men have had at least one experience in which they did not get or maintain an erection sufficient for intercourse. So the most feared male sexual problem is in fact an almost universal experience.

A common nonmedical cause of erectile dysfunction is trying to cope with PE by decreasing arousal to slow ejaculation. Approximately one in three men with PE also report erectile problems (Loudon 1988). The man feels caught between a rock and a hard place: if there is a lot of stimulation he will quickly ejaculate, but lack of stimulation results in erectile dysfunction. So the man rushes to intercourse because he fears losing his erection before he ejaculates.

Most men would prefer to take a medication like Viagra (sildenafil) or Cialis (tadalafil) to solve the erection problem, rather than address it with the partner. In fact, Viagra or Cialis can be a valuable resource by increasing blood flow to the penis and reducing performance anxiety. However, a pill cannot return the male to the easy, automatic, autonomous erections of his youth. The key to regaining erectile comfort and confidence is to relax, slow down and enjoy the pleasuring process, take in erotic sensations, and not rush intercourse or orgasm. It is crucial to be aware that the erection can wane but will become easily erect again if you stay relaxed and actively participate in the pleasuring and erotic process. You cannot be a "spectator" of your penis; sex is an involved, interactive experience.

Coexisting Sexual Problems in Women

Common female sexual problems that coexist with PE are *inhibited sexual desire* (acquired or lifelong), *difficulty reaching orgasm* (at all or during partner sex), *dyspareunia* (painful intercourse), *difficulty becoming aroused,* and *vaginismus* (constriction of the muscles of the vaginal opening making penetration for intercourse difficult or impossible). PE and female sexual dysfunction are often interrelated; one problem may contribute to the other. As a couple, you'll be most successful at improving your sexual relationship if you each take responsibility for communicating your needs and commit to working together as an intimate team.

The Resources section at the end of this book lists a number of excellent self-help sources for understanding and changing female sexual problems and dysfunction. If you desire more help, we recommend consultation with a credentialed sex therapist (see Choosing an Individual, Couple, or Sex Therapist for guidelines). Seeing a sex therapist is a sign of good judgment, not a sign that you are crazy or that this is an overwhelming problem. A professional therapist assesses the sexual problems and helps design a change program that addresses the female problem, male problem, and couple problem. Ongoing therapy helps the couple stay focused and motivated.

How You Can Best Use This Book

This book presents a state-of-the-art approach to PE, integrating new scientific research with the best, most comprehensive clinical practice. Our goal is to help men and couples understand and change the psychological, relational, medical, and situational factors that cause PE.

To benefit from our program, you'll need to take an active role by engaging in the self-tests and exercises. We urge both partners to be involved in the learning and change process, building awareness and skills. As you work together to improve ejaculatory control, you will enhance your sexual self-confidence and mutual enjoyment and satisfaction.

Each chapter builds on information in the previous chapters. The first three chapters include basic information and guidelines. Chapters 4 and 5 actively involve you in becoming aware of your personal type of PE and its impact on you and your relationship. Chapters 6, 7, and 8 are the core of the change process. We will help you carefully implement ejaculatory control strategies and techniques targeted for your particular type of PE. Chapter 9 will help you develop your unique couple sexual style. Chapter 10 presents a range of strategies and techniques to help you maintain sexual gains and prevent relapse. The more broad-based, flexible, and variable your approach to sex—including intercourse—the less vulnerable you are to relapse.

Be Patient and Use All Your Resources

PE is a complex problem with many causes and dimensions, but you can understand it and change it. For some couples, learning ejaculatory control will be a fairly easy process involving just one or two interventions, but most couples will need to use a number of techniques. Be aware that the change process is usually gradual and requires persistence, practice, and patience. It is important to remain motivated and focused and to use all your resources to address the factors involved in your PE.

These resources might include medical evaluation and treatment, medication, exercise, relaxation, several or all of the cognitive and behavioral techniques in this book, individual or couple therapy, improved communication and conflict resolution skills, increased emotional empathy, and time set aside for intimacy.

We congratulate you for having the courage and wisdom to address the problem of PE. We want you to feel empowered and motivated to resolve PE and enjoy the pleasures and satisfactions of couple sexuality.

2

Developing Realistic
Expectations about Sex

As an adolescent, John absorbed the idea that a real man is always ready for sex, no matter what the situation. John learned from sex magazines and from talking to his buddies that a man was supposed to be the sexual expert, and to have doubts or questions was to be a wimp. Like in porn videos, John was to have an erection at will, and his enormous penis would last as long as he wanted and satisfy the woman every time.

John could not live up to the image of the perfect sexual performer. John worried about penis size and about whether his desire and experiences were below normal. He felt inadequate, defensive, and guilty. He avoided serious conversations about sex. He felt that if his friends knew about his PE, they would make fun of him.

Likewise, John's girlfriend was filled with confusion and negative feelings. Did John care about her? She felt frustrated with the sex, resentful that John would not talk with her, and angry that sex did not get better. John and his partner were trapped in the miscommunication and myths perpetuated by the traditional male-female double standard.

To approach PE successfully, you'll need to take a critical look at these traditional views. It is especially important to challenge male performance myths, replacing these with positive, realistic expectations about the male body and couple sex. Part of the goal of PE treatment is for the man and his partner to have reasonable expectations about sex and sexual function within the context of an intimate relationship.

Understanding Your Body

To have control over when you ejaculate, you need to have an accurate and realistic understanding of your sexual physiology (how your sexual body works). In this chapter, we will explain in detail the physiology of male and female sexual response, especially the male ejaculation process. We will provide clear information about sexual desire, arousal, and orgasm. We will take a closer look at female desire and arousal and how this relates to PE. Then we'll guide you through evaluating your sexual expectations, sharing them with your partner, and working together to align your expectations.

Anatomy and Physiology of Sexual Response and Ejaculation

You may, at first thought, not be interested in the mechanics of ejaculation. But you'll find that accurate knowledge about your sexual body gives you an appreciation of why strategies like whole-body physical relaxation, conscious focus on pleasure, and pelvic muscle relaxation can be helpful in developing ejaculatory control. Accurate knowledge will also help you accept your body and its workings without resentment and frustration.

The Human Sexual Response Cycle

In 1966, Masters and Johnson revolutionized the human sexuality field by describing four stages of the sexual response cycle: *excitement, plateau, orgasm,* and *resolution.* Not only did they describe what happened during sexual arousal and orgasm, they measured physiological changes in blood flow and neurological response. In 1974, psychiatrist Helen Kaplan broadened the Masters and Johnson model to include an initial stage, *sexual desire.* Desire is associated with psychological and relational factors rather than solely focused on physiological factors.

The complete sexual response cycle consists of five phases: desire, excitement (arousal), plateau, orgasm, and satisfaction (resolution).

Desire. The desire phase involves sexual anticipation, fantasy, yearning, and both physical and emotional openness to sexual activity.

Excitement. During the excitement phase, in addition to a subjective sense of sexual pleasure, you experience erection, and a few droplets of secretions may appear from the tip of the penis. Women experience increased blood flow to the pelvis, vaginal lubrication, swelling in the external genitalia, narrowing of the outer third of the vagina, breast swelling, and lengthening and widening of the inner two-thirds of the vagina.

Plateau. The plateau phase is when the body's arousal levels off. If the body is physiologically relaxed, it will maintain pleasurable arousal without ejaculation or orgasm. This phase is limited or even nonexistent for you as a man with PE. During the plateau phase, the body "settles in" (becomes saturated with pleasure). Unless there is continuing stimulation of your penis, it is normal for your erection to go down or "take a break." Not understanding that this is normal, men unnecessarily panic, thinking that they have "lost" their erection and fearing it will never come back. This panic is a huge distraction, which disrupts the plateau phase, and indeed the erection, which is then difficult to regain. But with calm relaxation and trust in your body, all that is required is direct gentle touch to the penis and your erection will easily come back from "break."

The plateau phase is especially important for you to understand because it is the platform for ejaculatory control. There are two parts of this phase, excitement toleration and excitement saturation. By becoming skilled at techniques based in the plateau phase, you can enjoy pleasure and solidify ejaculatory control.

Orgasm. Sexual pleasure peaks during the orgasm phase and is accompanied by rhythmic contraction of the pelvic muscles and the release of sexual tension. In men, a sensation of ejaculatory inevitability precedes the contractions that result in ejaculation. In women, contractions occur in the outer third of the vaginal wall.

Satisfaction. During the satisfaction phase, the body gradually returns to the nonaroused state. Both the man and woman experience a pleasant afterglow, feeling relaxed and sexually satisfied. The length of the satisfaction or physical resolution phase is related to the length of the arousal and plateau phases. With PE, because lovemaking is brief, your erection will go down quickly after ejaculation. As you learn more relaxed arousal and extended plateau lovemaking, your penis will only go down halfway after ejaculation and remain so for a while. For most men, this provides the option to continue intercourse after a brief rest (perhaps thirty seconds) even though the penis is not as hard as before. Intercourse during the satisfaction phase can feel close and pleasing.

After ejaculation, men are temporarily unable to regain an erection and achieve orgasm, but women can respond almost immediately to additional stimulation. For men, this period when the body cannot sexually respond again—the *refractory* period—varies with age from almost unnoticed for a seventeen-year-old, to thirty to sixty minutes for a man in midlife, to a day or two for a sixty- to eighty-year-old man.

Ejaculation Physiology

To understand our approach to PE, you'll need to know more about how ejaculation works. The process of ejaculation involves several events: *erection, emission, ejaculation,* and *orgasm.* These processes are integrated by a complex set of interactions between the neurological system, hormonal system, and vascular system that combine to create a smooth chain of physiological events.

Erection refers to the events in the brain, nervous system, and vascular system leading to penile rigidity.

Emission refers to the collection and transport of fluids from several glands inside your groin that form the semen in preparation for ejaculation. Sperm from your testicles travel through a small tube called the *vas deferens,* which joins up in your *prostate gland* with the tube exiting your *bladder* to form your *urethra* tube. Then your urethra (the same tube that carries urine) runs through your chestnut-sized prostate, then down and out through your penis.

With arousal, the neck or exit of the bladder closes (that is why it is difficult to urinate when you are aroused and have an erection), your testicles are drawn up against your body, and semen collects in the *verumontanum,* a balloonlike chamber inside the prostate gland. When you get so excited that you are about to ejaculate, the verumontanum fills with semen, enlarging to three times its normal size. This pressure triggers the sensation of ejaculatory inevitability and the reflex of ejaculation.

Technically, ejaculatory control is actually emission control because once emission occurs you will ejaculate within seconds. This is why we teach you how to work with your body to enjoy more pleasure, and why we encourage you to just enjoy the pleasure of ejaculation once you feel that it is inevitable. Consider a space shuttle launch. The countdown proceeds to "five, four, three, two, one, ignition . . . ," and several seconds later the mission control announcer declares, ". . . and we have liftoff." Once ignition occurs, there is no stopping the launch; it will take off. From your sexual body's perspective, ignition is emission, with the feeling of ejaculatory inevitability, and liftoff is ejaculation, with the feeling of orgasm.

Ejaculation is the process of pushing the seminal fluids out of the "balloon" (verumontanum) inside the prostate through the urethra and out of the penis. Ejaculation occurs when a critical level of nerve input from the pressure of the verumontanum reaches the spinal cord and causes the reflexive ejaculatory response. The pelvic muscles are directly involved in ejaculation by rhythmically contracting to force the semen out, so consciously relaxing them can assist you in learning ejaculatory control. In chapter 8 you'll learn how to identify and relax these muscles as one of the PE management techniques.

Orgasm refers to the subjective experience of pleasure associated with ejaculation. Orgasm is a natural, healthy extension of the pleasuring-arousal-intercourse process. Orgasm and ejaculation are usually experienced as one and the same, although physiologically they are two distinct processes. Orgasm is primarily an experience in the brain. Though emission, ejaculation, and orgasm are integrated events and seem simultaneous, technically, erection is not required for ejaculation and ejaculation is not required for orgasm because they are controlled by separate neurological mechanisms.

Ejaculation Neurology

How the nervous system (*neurophysiology*) brings about ejaculation is only partially understood. *Selective serotonin reuptake inhibitor* (SSRI) medications affect the level of serotonin in the neurologic system, suppressing ejaculation. In chapter 6 we describe medications that can slow ejaculation.

With sexual activity, sensations are conveyed from your genitals through the nerves deep in your abdomen and from there to the spinal cord. These impulses stimulate reflexes in the spinal cord or ascend the spinal cord to your brain.

While ejaculation is technically a biological reflex involving the verumontanum in the prostate, your brain is very much involved in the process. You interpret sensual information, which may either augment ("turn on") or inhibit ("turn off") your arousal, and your brain responds with signals sent down to your lower spinal cord. From there, the impulse links up with neurologic impulses from your verumontanum to signal your ejaculatory system, which results in emission. At the same time, nerve signals are sent to stimulate your *pelvic floor muscles* (the *bulbocavernosus, ischiocavernosus,* and *pubococcygeus* muscles), resulting in those two to ten rhythmic contractions characteristic of ejaculation.

This kind of basic knowledge about your body can help you understand features of our comprehensive program. For example, notice that your brain plays an "interpreter" role in your arousal and influences ejaculation. You can help regulate your ejaculation by managing your mental focus during arousal using cognitive ejaculation control or "pacing" techniques that we will teach you (*entrancement arousal, the arousal continuum*). Also appreciate that the pelvic muscles are the muscles of ejaculation, and you can help regulate your ejaculation by learning to relax these muscles during sexual excitement. We will teach you these techniques in chapter 8.

Reconsidering Your Expectations of Your Sexual Body

Now that you've read about the physiological process for ejaculation, do you think your sexual expectations were grounded on accurate knowledge of your body? What ideas did you have that may have created unrealistic expectations of your body's sexual performance? Does understanding the ejaculatory process help you accept your amazing body as well as its limitations? How open are you to replacing your old ideas with new, realistic expectations?

The Integrated Model of Sexuality

It is important to remember that sex is more than your penis, intercourse, and ejaculation. Sexuality is an integral, positive part of you as a man, and includes your attitudes, emotions, behavior, body image, physical well-being, values, and—most important—how you feel about your relationship. At its essence, sexuality is an interpersonal process. Although males and females have very different sexual socialization as adolescents, men and women have many more sexual similarities than differences as adults. Both you and your partner can value sexuality as individuals and as a couple.

The integrated biopsychosocial model of sexual response involves desire, arousal, orgasm, and satisfaction. Arousal and orgasm have little enduring value unless you experience desire and satisfaction, individually and as a couple. This broader concept of sexuality is important to our program for understanding and changing PE. We believe that sexuality is best understood and treated as a couple issue. Even if you currently do not have a sexual partner, notice that your mind will imagine a partner, react to a partner from your past, or wish to meet that special woman in the near future. Even without a partner now, you are in a sexual relationship in your mind.

Female Sexual Desire and PE

Part of being realistic about sexual expectations is accurately understanding female sexual desire and arousal. Physician Rosemary Basson (2001) has outlined a new model for women's sexual arousal. She notes that in the beginning phase of a new relationship, romantic love and passionate sex lead to easy sexual response for women, but in a long-term relationship (after one or more years), increased distractions and fatigue lead to a different kind of sexual response.

Basson depicts healthy female sexual response in an established relationship as follows: Women begin in sexual neutrality, but sensing an emotional need to be sexual, an opportunity to be sexual, her partner's desire, or an awareness of one or more potential benefits that are important to her and the relationship (for example, emotional closeness, bonding, love, affection, healing, acceptance, or commitment), she may choose to move from sexual neutrality to seeking sensual contact and stimulation. With beginning sexual arousal, she may become aware at that time of desire to continue the experience for sexual reasons and experience more arousal which may or may not include wanting orgasm. This arousal level brings her a sense of physical well-being with the added pleasure of spin-offs such as emotional closeness, bonding, love, affection, and acceptance.

In this new model, women have a lower biological urge for the release of sexual tension than men. Rather, women's motivation to have sex stems from a number of potential gains that are not strictly sexual but are additions to the physical pleasure. Women's sexual arousal is greatly influenced by subjective mental excitement. Orgasmic release is not necessary for satisfaction; it does not occur at each sexual encounter.

Women's sexual desire is often a responsive rather than a spontaneous event. It develops after initial sensual contact. While a man's sexual desire may be energized by physical drive, typically a woman's sexual desire develops from her receptivity to gentle, relaxed sensual touching. This touching leads down the path to sexual desire and continues to emotional closeness, affection, sensuality, and eroticism.

Understanding Your Partner's Reaction to PE

This view of a woman's sexual response offers an understanding of why many women eventually become frustrated, hurt, or angry at experiencing PE lovemaking. Not only is the sensual value of sex frustrated, but more importantly the intimacy potential is sabotaged. This is exacerbated when the man stops lovemaking because of his frustration, apologizes, and "goes away" emotionally or physically after ejaculating.

This understanding of your partner's sexual response can help you both become more accepting and respectful of each other's sexual experience. This gives you context and motivation for learning to control ejaculation. You especially can learn to respond differently when you ejaculate before you want. Too often, men mistakenly think that PE is a sexual frustration for the woman rather than an emotional intimacy frustration. It is less about your sexual performance and more about shared closeness and emotional intimacy.

Developing Realistic Sexual Expectations

To learn ejaculatory control, you need to pilot yourself with realistic expectations. You can't expect more of your body than it is biologically built to do. We've already looked at some of the myths about male and female sexuality. Now let's take a look at your own expectations about sex.

EXERCISE: EVALUATING YOUR SEXUAL EXPECTATIONS

What do you expect about your sexual life? How does this compare to what actually goes on with other couples? What are positive, realistic expectations? Consider what we know about couple sexuality from clinical observations and scientific studies. At the beginning of each section, ask yourself what your expectations are. If you are part of a couple, ask your partner to do this exercise too. Write down your responses.

Frequency

How often do you expect to have sex? What influences this: the quality of your relationship, your body's urge, the balance of work and leisure time? Do you and your partner agree on frequency? What does it mean if you are having less, or more, sex than you expect?

The average sexual frequency for married couples is between four times a week and once every two weeks. Contrary to popular belief, married couples are more sexually active and satisfied than couples who are dating or living together. For couples in their twenties, average intercourse frequency is two to three times a week, and for couples in their fifties, it is once a week (Michael et al. 1994). Couples who are sexual less than twice a month may find it hard to develop and maintain ejaculatory control. You'll have the most success with ejaculatory control if you establish a regular rhythm of being sexual.

Length

How long should sex last? What is the relationship between time and quality? How long should intercourse last? One minute? Five minutes? Thirty minutes? An hour? What does length of sex mean for you?

The typical lovemaking encounter lasts from fifteen to forty-five minutes, which includes two to seven minutes of intercourse (Leiblum and Rosen 1989). A sexual encounter can vary from a two-minute quickie to an intimate, sensual, erotic two-hour experience. Lovemaking includes verbal and nonverbal communication, pleasuring, intercourse, and afterplay. Contrary to media myths and male braggadocio, few intercourse experiences involve ten minutes or longer of thrusting. These figures shock most men and women.

Arousal

In what situations do you find it easy to get an erection (men)/become lubricated (women)? When is it more difficult? What does it mean when you have difficulty getting an erection/becoming lubricated? What does it mean when your erection/lubrication wanes before or during intercourse?

Whether arousal failure happens once every ten times, once a month, or once a year, it is normal to occasionally not have an erection or lubrication sufficient for intercourse (remember that it's also normal for your erection/lubrication to "take a break" during the plateau phase). When this occurs, rather than panicking and feeling you are back at square one, you can just continue with erotic, nonintercourse sex to orgasm for one or both of you.

Ejaculatory Control

What is a realistic expectation about ejaculatory control? How have you determined this? What does it mean if you ejaculate fast? How much control are you supposed to have over ejaculation? Whose responsibility is it to "time" ejaculation?

What about PE specifically? How do you know when you are "cured"? What does it mean to have "reasonable" choice over when to be orgasmic? What is a realistic expectation about orgasm for the woman?

One key is to maintain the focus on sharing pleasure during intercourse. In other words, if you're both satisfied with the pleasure you're giving and receiving, ejaculatory control will matter less.

Another key is seeing intercourse as a mutual, interactive experience. Most men find it relatively easy to identify the point of ejaculatory inevitability and to learn slowing down and ejaculatory control with manual and oral stimulation. Ejaculatory control during intercourse is more challenging because it requires more cooperation and interaction.

Satisfaction

What do you require to feel sexually and emotionally satisfied? Must you ejaculate? Should every sexual encounter be equally satisfying? Why is a poor sexual experience distressing for you? Do you think that "mercy sex" (only pleasing your partner) is okay? Complete the sentence, "I am wonderfully sexually satisfied when . . ."

Even among well-functioning, satisfied married couples, half or fewer of their experiences are equally satisfying to both partners. In fact, if the couple has one or two experiences a month of movie-quality sex, they can count themselves as very fortunate. Perhaps 20 to 25 percent of sexual experiences are very good for one partner (usually the man) and good for the other. Another 20 to 25 percent of sexual experiences are okay but not remarkable. The most important thing to understand is that 5 to 15 percent of sexual experiences are mediocre, dissatisfying, or dysfunctional (Frank, Anderson, and Rubenstein 1978). Remember, this is true of well-functioning, satisfied couples.

EXERCISE: NEGOTIATING REASONABLE SEXUAL EXPECTATIONS WITH YOUR PARTNER

Now that you've each examined your own expectations, you'll want to compare your expectations as a couple and try to come to a flexible consensus that fits your relationship. This can be a difficult process! Take your time. Do your best to remain open-minded and communicate respectfully. It is normal and even healthy to have differences. If you find that your expectations are very different or you're having trouble communicating, you may want to seek help from a therapist.

1. How often do you expect to have sex? Why is this frequency important to you? Where does your sexual desire come

from? What is a comfortable frequency for you as a couple that fits your lifestyle?

2. How long do you expect foreplay (pleasuring) to last? Intercourse? Why is this length of time meaningful to you? Can you agree on a range of time that is comfortable for you both?

3. How comfortable are you accepting that it is normal for a man's erection or a woman's lubrication to come and go during a relaxed sexual interaction?

4. What do you consider a good range of time for you to have intercourse? How long do you like the slow, sensual intercourse? How long the more intense intercourse? What is your wish for varying the pace of intercourse?

5. In what percent of encounters should you choose when to ejaculate?

6. In what percent of encounters should the woman have an orgasm? How?

7. What determines your satisfaction with your sexual interaction?

8. What percent of the time do you expect sex should be great, what percent satisfactory, what percent all right, and what percent poor quality? What do you think is reasonable?

9. How do you each want to handle times when sex goes poorly?

Steve and Suzanne's Story

Steve and Suzanne had been a couple for six years, married for four years, and had an eighteen-month-old son. They agreed sex was best in the early months of the relationship. The excitement of finding each other, developing their relationship, experiencing romantic love, and having new and exciting sex added a special charge to their lives. Steve had lifelong PE, but the frequency of sex and the enthusiasm of their romantic relationship made the ejaculatory problem seem unimportant. Suzanne felt attracted to Steve, attractive and cared for by Steve, and very excited to be in this relationship. She naively hoped that with time the quality of intercourse would improve, but was not upset by the rapid ejaculation. Steve enjoyed second intercourse opportunities where his control was somewhat better. He found Suzanne's passion and enthusiasm a real turn-on.

Steve was happy with Suzanne, their marriage, and their family. Steve just ignored the PE problem. Some men find that with increased sexual comfort and experience, ejaculatory control gradually improves without their needing to do anything specific. However, for most men, PE becomes a chronic sexual problem, which is what happened with Steve.

Suzanne eventually became frustrated and then sexually turned off. At first she tried to raise the issue of intercourse quality indirectly and tactfully, but Steve just ignored her or treated the dissatisfaction as her problem.

Finally the issue exploded into a nasty argument after a sexual encounter. Suzanne complained that Steve was so quick and selfish. He accused Suzanne of being a whiner and frigid person. Having an argument about sex when they were naked and emotionally vulnerable felt awful, but they couldn't seem to stop themselves. Their conversation quickly degenerated into hurt, defensiveness, and anger. Steve felt unfairly attacked, and Suzanne felt Steve was mean and had no desire to improve their sexual life.

Steve stewed about this for two days and then decided he would "show" Suzanne. Without telling her, he made an appointment at a male sex clinic which advertised on sports radio. Steve received medication which was to delay his orgasm. Without saying anything to Suzanne, he became obsessed with the goal of getting Suzanne to have an orgasm before he ejaculated. Sex became a crucial test of Steve's manhood: he had to hold out until she had an orgasm.

At first, Suzanne was pleased that Steve seemed more caring and intercourse was lasting longer, but then she became turned off by Steve's obsessive focus on her orgasm. She began to dread and resent sex. Suzanne's desire and arousal was much reduced, which further frustrated Steve, and he became even more defensive. Sex was no longer an intimate, sharing experience; instead it was a struggle over orgasm. The relationship was dispirited, sinking under the weight of misunderstanding and performance pressure. Steve was being his own worst enemy, and Suzanne was feeling increasingly alienated and turned off.

It was Suzanne who made the call to a couple therapist with a subspecialty in sex therapy. This was a very wise move. Steve and Suzanne were ideal candidates for couple sex therapy because they had a genuine marital bond of respect, trust, and intimacy and a desire for a satisfying sexual relationship. The PE and sexual misunderstanding were draining intimacy and threatening to destabilize their marriage.

The first priority in therapy was to reinforce the importance of intimacy and pleasuring. Steve had misinterpreted Suzanne's comments as meaning that he was a terrible lover. With the help of the therapist, Steve was able to understand that Suzanne valued him as a loving, attractive husband and wanted to work with him to enhance their sexual life so that the marriage was satisfying and secure. Her request was that Steve be a more sensitive, slower lover. Suzanne was not demanding that Steve be a perfect sexual performer but a more involved, caring lover.

Suzanne had a variable arousal and orgasm pattern. She enjoyed being orgasmic with manual and oral stimulation as well as during intercourse. She did want Steve to develop better ejaculatory control, but more importantly, she wanted Steve to be willing to engage in additional erotic stimulation during intercourse. Steve needed to affirm that he was learning ejaculatory control for himself and the relationship, not to perform for Suzanne. With this new understanding, they decided to work together on developing ejaculatory control.

At times, Steve and Suzanne found the ejaculatory control exercises tedious, and change was slow, but as long as they continued to communicate and cooperate, it was enjoyable. Suzanne felt that she had an integral role in the exercises and that her emotional and sexual feelings were important. Steve felt that Suzanne was an intimate ally and that her desire and arousal enhanced the sexual experience. As he came to understand and appreciate the nuances of desire, arousal, orgasm, and satisfaction for himself and for Suzanne, the sexual relationship and PE improved. As a bonus, Steve and Suzanne expanded their repertoire of pleasuring and erotic techniques. Both learned to be sexually assertive, express intimate feelings, enjoy prolonged intercourse, see orgasm as a voluntary process, and enjoy flexible, variable sexual experiences.

What You Can Expect from Our Program for Change

In the same way that it's important to have reasonable expectations of yourself and your body, it's important to know what you can reasonably expect from our approach to PE. You won't become a sexual machine that can last for hours and hours. You *will* learn ejaculatory control and enjoy arousal during prolonged intercourse. You will enhance your relationship by learning to enjoy and share the entire sexual experience: intimacy, pleasuring, eroticism, arousal, intercourse, and afterplay.

Learning ejaculatory control is like learning any skill. It is a gradual process requiring feedback and practice. You'll need to approach this as a team. After all, an interested, involved sexual partner is the best aphrodisiac! You and your partner need to utilize all of your resources to learn and maintain ejaculatory control.

The essence of ejaculatory control involves learning to carefully attend to your body's physical sensations, relaxing your body while aroused, identifying the point of ejaculatory inevitability, maintaining awareness of pleasurable sensations at high levels of arousal, and having reasonable (not perfect) control over when you will let go and orgasm. It involves cognitive, behavioral, and emotional skills; it is not a mechanical process.

Many men find it easier to develop awareness, comfort, and skills with self-stimulation. Practicing ejaculatory control during partner sex, especially intercourse, is more complex and challenging, but if you can do it by yourself, you can learn to do it during partner sex.

Like Steve and Suzanne, you and your partner can expect to develop greater intimacy and a more satisfying sex life. It's hard work, but it's worth it!

3

Understanding the Causes and Effects of PE

Real-life problems are rarely simple, easy to solve, or magically fixed, in spite of quick-fix promises. The major reason traditional treatments of PE have failed to help so many is that PE is not a simple problem with a simple cure. While the experience of PE is pretty much the same for all men—quick and uncontrolled ejaculation—there are actually nine different types of PE, each with a different cause. PE may be a physical problem, involving the neurological system, medical illness, physical injuries, or side effects of drugs. It may be psychological or interpersonal, stemming from personality characteristics, unresolved issues from your family of origin or personal history, anxieties and stressors, relationship stresses, or sexual skills deficits.

It's not just the causes of PE that are complicated—the effects are complicated too. PE can have a devastating impact on your self-esteem, your sex life, and your relationship. These effects, in turn, can make PE worse. It's a vicious cycle.

In this chapter, we'll look at the nine different types of PE: four physical, four psychological or relational, and one mixed type involving another sexual dysfunction. Then we'll focus on the psychological and relational causes and effects, because these are the aspects that you have the most control over. The psychological and relational causes are particularly complex and intertwining, so we'll offer you a model to help you understand how these dimensions fit together. In chapter 4 we'll help you determine which type or types of PE you have. Then you'll be prepared to develop a comprehensive and effective approach to managing your PE.

Possible Causes of PE

Scientific research helps us to sort out myths from reality. When it comes to PE, this difference is very important.

Neurologic System PE

Neurologic system PE is caused by a physiological predisposition in the nervous system to ejaculate quickly. As you'll remember from chapter 2, ejaculation is triggered by a reflex. Montreal psychiatrist Pierre Assalian (1988) states that some men with PE have a "constitutionally hypersensitive sympathetic nervous system" (p. 215)—in other words, a very quick reflex. This type of PE occurs throughout a man's life, with every partner, and in all sexual situations, including masturbation.

Historically, this was the predominant explanation of PE. Rapid ejaculation was believed to be normal and even to provide an evolutionary advantage. Kinsey, Pomeroy, and Martin (1948) noted that 75 percent of men ejaculated in less than two minutes of intercourse. Researchers including Bixler (1986) and Hong (1984) assumed that human behavior is similar to animal behavior and noted that the "top dog" or "alpha" animal ejaculates quickly. Hong observed that the normal pattern for most primates is to ejaculate within three to ten seconds of intercourse. Many professionals concluded from their clinical impressions that PE must have physiological origins. For example, urologist Schapiro's classic report published in 1943 attributes PE to neurologic efficiency.

More recently, researchers have theorized that genetic inheritance plays some role in the lifelong physiological predisposition to ejaculate quickly. Waldinger (1998) found that 91 percent of men with lifelong PE also had a first relative with lifelong PE. Rowland (1999) found physiological differences between PE and non-PE males. For example, men with PE have a faster *bulbocavernosus reflex* (that is, a faster neurological response in the pelvic muscles).

Physical Illness PE

Physical illnesses may cause PE. Here the PE is acquired, not lifelong, and occurs in all sexual situations. A number of acute diseases are known to affect ejaculation speed. Some are common illnesses, such as urinary tract infection, while others are very rare. The illness that most frequently causes PE is *prostatitis* (prostate infection), although virtually any urologic illness may have this effect.

Physical Injury PE

Some cases of PE are caused by temporary or permanent physical damage to the body that directly or indirectly affects ejaculatory mechanisms. Because of the injury, the neurological connection with the genital area is compromised so that at least some sensation and control of ejaculation is impaired or lost.

Drug Side-Effect PE

PE may occur as the result of use of or withdrawal from certain chemical agents. This type of PE is acquired and occurs in all sexual situations. Examples include withdrawal from certain tranquilizers or opiates, or even use of over-the-counter cold medications like Sudafed (pseudoephedrine).

Psychological System PE

Psychological system PE is caused by chronic psychological disorders such as bipolar mood disorder (sometimes called manic depression), obsessive-compulsive disorder, chronic depression, generalized anxiety disorder, schizophrenia, personality disorder (for example, avoidant personality disorder, dependent personality disorder, or borderline personality disorder), post-traumatic stress disorder (the aftereffects of witnessing tragedy or being victimized), or developmental disorders such as attention deficit/hyperactivity disorder. It may also be caused by the ongoing psychological effects of alcoholism or drug abuse, or by chronic, unresolved personal issues.

While significant psychological problems may cause PE, the vast majority of men with PE do not have major psychological problems. There is no common personality profile for men with psychological system PE. This type of PE typically occurs throughout a man's life and in all sexual situations.

Psychological Distress PE

Psychological distress PE is caused by temporary psychological difficulties such as an adjustment disorder (temporary depression or anxiety), serious unusual stress, or acute depression. Psychological distress may also result from PE, for example, when physical illness PE causes psychological distress. While there is no typical psychological profile for men with PE, the scientific literature reports that PE is more likely when the man has situational anxiety, reactive depression, loss of confidence, mistrust, frustration, anger, restrictive religious beliefs, negative feelings about his body and sexuality, or unrealistic expectations of sexual performance, or when he experiences internal conflicts such as between the roles of lover and father. Psychosocial stresses (for example, occupational stress, the death of a friend or parent, financial problems, or acculturation problems) may precipitate PE. Sometimes it is difficult to determine which is the chicken and which is the egg; it may be unclear whether the anxiety is the cause or result of PE. Psychological distress PE is acquired.

Men tend to underestimate the effect that psychological stress may have on their sexual functioning. The thinking goes something like this: "When there is such a profound problem as PE, the cause must be profound as well." But in fact, it does not take much psychological distress to disrupt sexual functioning.

Relationship Distress PE

Complicated interpersonal dynamics may cause PE or result from it. Relationship distress PE is rooted in interpersonal dynamics such as failure to communicate, hurtful misunderstandings, fear of romantic success, unresolved emotional conflicts, hypersensitivity to your partner, profound discomfort with or fear of intimacy, or other distresses such as mistrust in response to infidelity.

In short, general relationship deficiencies undermine the mutual emotional acceptance that is important to healthy sexual functioning. Even when PE is caused by something other than relationship distress, it can cause considerable damage to your relationship. Relationship distress PE is commonly acquired and limited to sex with the partner.

While there is no single interaction pattern among couples facing PE, there are several common patterns.

- The man is hypersensitive to his partner, fears failing and disappointing her, and is frequently self-blaming and apologetic. The woman is either shy and compliant or direct and aggressive.

- The man is self-absorbed and aloof from his partner's concerns. He may defend his dysfunction as a normal physiological response, while she may feel emotionally ignored and abandoned, and respond contentiously.

- The couple experiences unresolved relationship conflicts accompanied by perceived rejection, blaming, and criticism. They may struggle with the balance of autonomy and couple cohesion, empathy deficits, or a conflict-resolution impasse. One partner may feel abandoned by the other and take an avoidant or hostile stance. The PE may be a reciprocal and interactive problem that has more to do with relationship distress than sex itself.

- A sexual problem like PE serves as a surrogate problem, providing a focus for the couple's anxiety and dissatisfaction so that the rest of the relationship can remain functional. Sex might feel like the only relationship problem, but it is not.

- The man's PE coexists with a sexual dysfunction in the woman. Some women experience inhibited arousal, while others experience difficulty achieving orgasm in part because of their partner's PE. In other cases, her sex dysfunction interacts with his PE. For example, because of her inhibited desire, she may encourage him to "get it over with." If she experiences discomfort or pain during intercourse, he may hurry to limit the discomfort. In still other cases of acquired PE, the man's fast ejaculation may be a reaction to the woman's psychological distress (for example, anxiety or depression), or to her negative attitude toward sex, general discomfort with a sexual behavior (for example, oral sex), low sexual arousal, or inhibited orgasm.

Psychosexual Skills Deficit PE

Psychosexual skills deficit PE typically results from the man not having accurate and sufficient knowledge about his body, his partner's body, and sexual physiology (how sexual response works); holding unreasonable expectations about sexual performance; and lacking essential sensual skills to manage his body during sexual arousal. Some men also lack dating or interpersonal skills. This type of PE is lifelong but may not occur with masturbation.

Most men with psychologically caused PE usually have some limitations in psychosexual skills, if only to compensate for individual stresses or relationship tensions that rob sexuality of its natural bonding and emotional-healing capacity. In such cases the man has difficulty focusing on his own sensations; becomes preoccupied with anticipating failure; has difficulty relaxing his body while sexually aroused; lacks awareness of techniques for managing PE or uses ineffective techniques like distraction; focuses excessively on his partner's body and reactions; experiences restricted, uneasy, or anxious sensuality; or entertains distorted thoughts ("sex must be spontaneous" or "emotions are not involved in sex").

PE with Another Sexual Dysfunction (Mixed PE)

PE that coexists with another sexual dysfunction such as low sexual desire or erectile dysfunction occurs about one-third of the time and can reflect a complicated combination of physical and psychological causes. For example, a vascular cause for erectile dysfunction may combine with psychological and relationship distress that adds to PE. PE is sometimes caused by the man's efforts to compensate for a fear of erectile dysfunction. Treating the erectile dysfunction can, in turn, help resolve the PE. On the other hand, some men try so hard to halt PE that they unintentionally cause erectile dysfunction, which then leads to inhibited sexual desire.

The Multiple Dimensions of PE

In addition to understanding the multiple causes of PE, it is valuable to appreciate that PE is also *multidimensional*—that not only is there rarely one cause of PE, there is an interaction between the biological, medical, psychological, relational, and situational dimensions. For example, a prostate infection (medical) may interact with your self-esteem (psychological), affect communication with your partner (relational), and even influence your feelings about work and home life (psychological and situational). This intermingling and intertwining of the facets of our personalities and lives is normal. This is partly why PE can feel so confusing, so difficult to sort out. Yes, PE is complex.

To illustrate these dimensional interactions, consider Robert's effort to understand his PE. We identify some of the interacting dimensions in parentheses.

Robert's Story

Robert was thirty-four years old and had been married for eight years. He thought that he had a pretty good life: a happy marriage to Tonya, a five-year-old son, and a good career as a teacher. After several years of what he considered "okay" sexual performance, he began to ejaculate very quickly—within one minute. He felt perplexed (psychological). He began to feel irritated with his penis as he intended to last longer but his body seemed to betray him (biological and psychological). He was confused, sensing the chaos of trying to figure it out so he could do something about it (psychological). He tried to be aware and sensitive to Tonya, even felt hypersensitive to her actions, moods, and words, especially since she had recently said she was "less interested in sex" (psychological and relational). Since his PE developed after a long period of performing okay, he thought that maybe there was something wrong with his body (biological, medical). Should he see his doctor? But he hated going to his physician (psychological). He was almost phobic about blood draws (psychological and biological).

He realized too that he was very down and anxious (psychological) about the whole sex thing. None of his efforts to slow down ejaculation had helped. He was puzzled to notice that one time recently when he drank too much, he was able to last a little longer before ejaculating. Was alcohol an answer (biological)? He could not let himself go that route (psychological). Another time he lasted a little longer was when he had a sinus infection and had trouble breathing (biological).

Robert realized he was beginning to withdraw from sex and from Tonya (relational) but felt trapped, like he couldn't win (psychological). Even at work he noticed he sometimes could not concentrate well and felt distracted (relational, psychological). He also noticed, at times, that he was impatient with his son (psychological and relational). These things seemed to arise from his tension over the PE (psychological). What is this chaos? What to do?

With the help of assessment and intervention strategies and exercises, Robert and Tonya were able to understand and resolve his PE. You can do it, too.

You Can Understand Your PE

All of these aspects—biological/medical, psychological, relational, situational—interact in your effort to figure out your PE and change it. Without some organizational model, the chaos feels overwhelming. We will help you sort it out, make sense of it, see what you are up against, and figure out what you can do. If your case is simple, we are very happy for you. If your case is multidimensional like most, welcome aboard. We want to help you honestly see PE for the complex problem it is, use this deeper understanding to overcome the feeling of being overwhelmed and hopeless, and help you and your partner cooperate to improve your sexual life and relationship.

The Psychological and Relational Dimensions of PE

To help you understand the psychological and relationship aspects of PE, we offer you a framework, the *cognitive-behavioral-emotional* (CBE) model. This will help you make sense of the otherwise confusing experience of PE and organize your couple approach to overcoming PE.

The Cognitive-Behavioral-Emotional Model

The CBE model recognizes that each individual is composed of *cognitions,* or thoughts; *behaviors,* or actions; and *emotions,* or feelings. We'll describe these components, then show you how they are involved in your PE.

These dimensions of the CBE model interact almost automatically—thoughts influencing feelings, feelings influencing behaviors, and behaviors prompting thoughts and feelings. In the integrative CBE model, each component is valued and promotes change. Your insight will be strengthened by understanding the cognitions, behaviors, and emotions that constitute PE.

Cognitions or Thoughts

Cognitions involve ideas, beliefs, observations, interpretations, and reasoning. Psychologists Norman Epstein and Donald Baucom (2002) describe five distinct cognitions that affect our relationships: assumptions, standards, perceptions, attributions (explanations), and expectancies (expectations). These are unique to each person. Such cognitions are beneficial or detrimental to you depending on their effects on your feelings and actions.

Behaviors or Actions

We make decisions to act (or not act) based upon our thoughts and feelings. Technically, action is always a choice or decision. The freedom to choose your behavior may be mitigated by thoughts and feelings, but responsible and mature living mandates accountability for your behavior. While feelings are not viewed as ethical (that is, not judged to be good or bad), behaviors are. Behaviors may be constructive or destructive depending on their effect on each individual and the relationship.

Emotions or Feelings

Emotions are chemical-electrical "energy" events or experiences in your body. You label this energy according to how you experience these physical sensations: fear, sadness, loneliness, panic, satisfaction, anger, worry, contentment, frustration, pleasure, irritability, excitement, anxiety, wonderment, confusion, shame, guilt, comfort, embarrassment, resentment, safety. Feelings are "motivators" that prompt, penalize, or reward action. Feelings are not themselves good or bad, right or wrong. Feelings influence the thoughts we have and the actions we take. Emotions can be positive or negative depending on how you subjectively experience them and how they influence your behavior.

Sherry and Alex's Story

To illustrate this model, consider Alex and Sherry's experience of PE. Be aware of their thoughts, actions, and feelings. To help you identify these, we will label cognitions as (C), behaviors as (B), and emotions as (E). You may find some features similar to your own experience.

Alex's chronic PE led Sherry to perceive (C) him as selfish and rejecting of her desires, and Sherry felt dismissed (E). Alex did not intend (C) to be selfish. Rather, he was deeply perplexed (C) at his performance "failure" (B) and feared disappointing Sherry (E). Yet his actions (B) after ejaculating quickly appeared (C) selfish to Sherry.

Here is an outline of what was happening. With fast ejaculation (B), Alex appeared to Sherry (C) to be sexually satisfied by his orgasm (B), but he typically stopped pleasuring (B) Sherry ("he rolls over and goes to sleep"). Alex felt frustrated with himself (E), focused on his failure (C), apologized (B) to Sherry for PE, and stopped lovemaking, became quiet or withdrawn, or even left their bed (B).

For several years, Sherry had experienced Alex's PE and observed him (C) failing to seek professional help (B). All of these actions (B) seemed to Sherry to be insensitive (C) to her wants and feelings, hurt her deeply (E), felt like an abandonment (E), and seemed hard to interpret as anything other than an incredible selfishness (C). Her hurt (E) sometimes manifested as complaints, criticisms, and other expressions of anger (B), even rage at times. With this, Alex thought he was betrayed (C), and he misunderstood (C) Sherry's lack of support (B) when he failed (C) to control his ejaculation (B), but was confused (C) about what to do (B). Everything that he tried (B) (distracting himself, masturbating before lovemaking) failed (C). He felt completely hopeless (E) and inadequate (C), and avoided Sherry (B). She believed she was abandoned (C) and ignored by Alex (B), and felt hurt and angry (E).

Alex and Sherry's story shows how these complex and detrimental cognitions, behaviors, and emotions serve to cause, maintain, or exacerbate PE, or may become the psychological effects of PE caused by other factors. Some examples of negative cognitions that can be involved in PE are "I am a failure," "I am sexually inadequate," or "He is just selfish." Negative behaviors include withdrawal from your partner, silence, blaming, or failing to talk constructively with each other about the problem. Detrimental emotions include frustration, anger, shame, or confusion. Identifying these negative dimensions is a step in the process of overcoming the anguish of PE. You can stop these patterns and change them to more reasonable cognitions, cooperative behaviors, and positive feelings.

Relationship Identity, Cooperation, and Intimacy

PE exists within a relationship, not in a vacuum. Understanding relationship dimensions can help you make sense of your distress and alert you to areas to repair or strengthen as you address PE. Let's look at the CBE model of relationship health.

Relationship Identity

Relationship identity refers to the cognitive life of your relationship, comprising the expectations that each of you brings to the relationship, the relevance of your personal history, and what your relationship means to each of you. For example, how do you balance each other's needs for individual autonomy and relationship cohesion? In healthy relationships, each individual benefits from the relationship, and the relationship benefits from the input of each individual.

Relationship Cooperation

Relationship cooperation refers to your behavioral interactions: how you communicate, work together in a balanced way, and mutually solve problems effectively. Your thoughts and feelings are hidden from each other unless you communicate them through a behavior—typically by sharing through discussion or nonverbal gestures. This is why communication is such an important part of couple sexual growth.

Relationship Intimacy

Relationship intimacy refers to your relationship's "climate" or quality of emotional bond. Intimacy describes the emotional, friendship, and sexual aspects of your relationship—feelings of affection, commitment, and closeness.

These relationship themes fundamentally determine relationship satisfaction.

PE and Sexual Relationship Identity, Cooperation, and Intimacy

To help you more fully appreciate the interrelated dimensions of your PE, we'll describe specific types of cognitions involved in sexual relationship identity, behaviors that make up sexual relationship cooperation, and emotions associated with sexual relationship intimacy. The CBE model of relationship health can help you focus on what to strive for, not simply what to stop or "get over" from the past. Remember that the context for overcoming PE is not simply to slow down your ejaculation, but to enhance your relationship identity, cooperation, and emotional intimacy.

PE and the Role of Cognitions: Sexual Relationship Identity

Your cognitions about PE comprise the sexual "meaning" of PE. Discovering your and your partner's meanings of sexuality and PE is an important element in understanding your sexual dissatisfaction. Does PE mean a limitation on pleasure? Shame? Failure? Alienation? Does sex mean duty? Perfect performance? Is it "dirty but exciting"? Disgusting? Or, does sex mean vulnerable sharing? Comfort? Gentleness and tenderness? Acceptance? Playfulness? Intimacy?

The subjective meaning that PE has for you and your partner is determined by these cognitions, and they influence your emotional experiences during sex. You and your partner can understand each other more fully by sharing your thoughts about PE and the meaning of sex. You can also begin to change your experience of PE by replacing negative thoughts with positive ones.

Detrimental and Beneficial Cognitions with PE

Following are some common detrimental thoughts that men and women have when PE is a significant problem. We also offer beneficial thoughts that can replace them to help you alter PE's meaning and help motivate your changes. Be aware that beneficial cognitions are grounded in accurate knowledge about sex.

Assumptions about sex are cognitions about the characteristics of intimate relationships that you accept as true without question and govern how you interact.

Detrimental Cognitions	Beneficial Cognitions
• Good sex means long intercourse.	• Good sex involves flexible ways to share pleasure which invites personal and relationship joys.
• Movie-type sex is normal.	• Movie sex portrays impulsive, perfect-performance sex. We are real lovers, not actors in a Hollywood movie!

Standards or beliefs are cognitions about the characteristics that you think your sexual partner or relationship should have, and the judgments you make. Examples of detrimental *versus* beneficial standards are:

Detrimental Cognitions	Beneficial Cognitions
• Sex should always be romantic.	• Sex is sometimes romantic, sometimes routine, sometimes joyful, sometimes monotonous, sometimes deeply meaningful. Sex is a healthy part of our couple style.
• We should have sex four times a week because I've heard that is normal for our age.	• The frequency of sex should conform to the realities of our lives and be mutually satisfying.

Perceptions about sex are your cognitive "selective focus." You notice only a part of the information available. Which part depends on your emotional state, level of fatigue, prior experiences in similar situations, and preexisting cognitions and perceptions about sex.

Detrimental Cognitions	Beneficial Cognitions
• When he ejaculates, he immediately apologizes and goes away physically and emotionally, and I am abandoned.	• His apology and withdrawal may signal that he feels deeply ashamed, sexually inadequate, a failure. I'll ask him to physically stay involved after intercourse for the closeness or to be satisfied by other ways than intercourse.

- She punishes me with her anger when I come fast.

- Her anger manifests her hurt, loneliness, or feelings of emotional abandonment. I will tell her that I want to understand her feelings and to lead the way with the program in this book.

Attributions are the causal explanations you have about your PE. The explanations reflect your understanding of and sense of control over sexual experiences.

Detrimental Cognitions

- He ejaculates so fast because he is selfish.

Beneficial Cognitions

- PE is more than selfishness. What must he be feeling? Perhaps anxious? Ashamed? Inadequate? Powerless? Betrayed by his body's fast ejaculation? Afraid I will go to someone else?

- She is so resistant or passive when having sex because she no longer loves me. I have ruined our marriage because of PE.

- Sex is only one aspect of our intimate relationship. I wonder if she is passive during lovemaking because she anticipates the touching will end when I ejaculate? When I ejaculate quickly, I will ask her if I can hold her and rest for a minute, and then pleasure her with my hands.

Expectancies are the automatic predictions about what is likely to occur: "if this, then that." When thinking about PE, this often includes expectations that you will fail.

Detrimental Cognitions

- If we try to have sex, it won't work because I'll ejaculate fast; it will be a disappointment, and she'll be angry.

Beneficial Cognitions

- I will ask her to be part of my effort to learn ejaculatory control and heal the pain in our relationship caused by PE.

- If I ask for what I want sexually (like oral sex or slower touch), he will get upset.

- I will ask him kindly—and not during sex—whether he would like me to offer suggestions about the kinds of touch I really enjoy.

Changing the Way You Think about PE

You can change the way you think about PE based on realistic expectations of yourself and your relationship. Research supports that your way of thinking is the most important factor for change and satisfaction. Your negative thoughts about PE function as a self-fulfilling prophecy. Identifying the detrimental and limiting cognitions that you and your partner may have adopted toward your PE, and replacing them with realistic and constructive ones, is a very useful change strategy.

EXERCISE: CHANGING YOUR THOUGHTS ABOUT PE

Take a moment to consider your cognitions about your sex life: your assumptions, beliefs, perceptions, explanations, and expectancies. Each of these thoughts reflects the meaning sex has for you. How do you want to reframe the meaning of sex for you and your partner? What is its role in your intimate relationship? Choose one or two thoughts that you think are the most detrimental. Write a positive alternative for each. When those negative thoughts arise, consciously shift to the positive thought. You can share your thoughts with each other to help understand each other better.

PE and the Role of Behaviors: Sexual Relationship Cooperation

Behaviors are the "bridge" between you and your partner. Your thoughts and feelings can only be accurately known to each other through your actions, verbal and nonverbal. To address PE, you and your partner must focus on cooperative behavior that moves you toward your goal.

When your PE is not constructively addressed, it manifests in negative behavior. For example, the man avoids sex to avoid disappointment, avoids talking about the problem, acts as though nothing is wrong, pressures his partner to have orgasm other ways than through intercourse, or makes love rigidly and mechanically as he tries desperately to control his ejaculation. The woman may push her lover away, say hurtful things, rush sex to get it over with to avoid further hurt and frustration, or place limitations or conditions on sex.

Relationship conflict may cause PE when unresolved disagreements or repeated negative interactions undermine emotional intimacy. PE may cause relationship conflict when it is chronic and ignored. On the other hand, mutually resolved relationship conflict enhances emotional and sexual intimacy. Ordinary conflict presents opportunities for couples to deepen their emotional and sexual intimacy. Differences or disagreements about sexual interaction are common and normal; the issue is how well you deal with them. PE is an example of a relationship cooperation challenge. With a positive, respectful, affirming process of conflict resolution, partners develop a deeper understanding of how the other thinks and feels, a greater sense of self-esteem, greater respect and admiration for each other, more confidence that future conflict can be resolved, and increased goodwill and comfort, which facilitates sexual desire.

Detrimental and Beneficial Behaviors with PE

There are detrimental behaviors that cause, maintain, or worsen PE, as well as beneficial behaviors that may ameliorate or help PE.

Detrimental Actions	Beneficial Actions
• Verbally criticizing your partner or your partner's behavior.	• Calmly and openly expressing your own feelings.
• Withdrawing from your partner.	• Staying, being present, disclosing your feelings, or expressing your intention to work together.
• Anticipating sexual "failure" and then avoiding initiating sex.	• Calmly talking with your partner and openly acknowledging the dilemma you feel.
• Acting aloof or cold.	• Showing warmth and interest in cooperating, requesting what you want in a positive way.
• Apologizing when you ejaculate fast.	• Asking your partner how you can be responsive to her sexual feelings and desires, and how you can please her.

- Expressing frustration at yourself and your partner.

- Reminding yourself that expressing frustration doesn't help, then refocusing and recommitting to enhancing sensual and sexual pleasure.

- Refusing to discuss the sexual problem.

- Talking calmly, sharing your feelings, describing the dilemma you face, and asking for cooperation to enrich your sexual relationship.

- Threatening an affair, separation, or divorce. This is truly poisonous behavior because threats create anxiety and polarize you as a couple.

- Expressing your desire to join together to solve your difficulty as a couple.

Changing the Way You Act about PE

These examples of injurious behaviors (whether intended or not) and more beneficial actions involving PE are changes you and your partner can implement. Identifying your contribution and seeing what constructive changes you need to make are essential to your success.

EXERCISE: CHANGING YOUR BEHAVIORS ABOUT PE

From the list above, choose at least one and up to three behaviors to focus on changing. If you slip into old detrimental behaviors, forgive yourself, then recommit to choosing more positive behaviors.

PE and the Role of Feelings: Sexual Relationship Intimacy

In the emotional life of your relationship, PE may bring about hurtful feelings (humiliation, rejection, loneliness, or abandonment) that undermine beneficial feelings (acceptance, closeness, and love). The emotional suffering of many couples with PE is quiet, hidden, and often deeply upsetting, which only adds to the confusion and sense of hopelessness.

Detrimental Emotions with PE

Common feelings for the man with PE are bewilderment, shame, disappointment, an intense sense of failure and inadequacy, self-doubt, loneliness, humiliation, frustration, hurt, depression, embarrassment, heightened performance anxiety, hopelessness, interpersonal alienation, and dread of talking about sex.

The woman may at first feel supportive and sympathetic and offer encouraging and affirming responses, but with chronic avoidance by the man, she may feel lonely, emotionally abandoned, resentful that he ignores the issue (by not talking about it and not seeking help), sad, confused, frustrated, rejected, or alienated. She may begin to dread sex as an ordeal to be endured.

Changing the Way You Feel about PE

Your goal as a couple is to transform these detrimental feelings into more constructive and beneficial ones: self-confidence, warmth, trust, comfort, closeness, calmness, understanding, love, empathy, mutual acceptance, specialness, safety, pleasure, playfulness, collaboration, and strength. Beginning to change your cognitions and behaviors about PE will help transform your feelings about PE.

The meaning of PE to each partner has substantial emotional significance. When the meaning of PE is hidden for you and your partner, or when you are reluctant or unable to discuss the distinctive meaning that PE has for you, it is very difficult to share the experience of change and cooperate. Identifying and understanding the meaning of PE provides an important foundation for you to accept your dilemma and begin to replace detrimental cognitions, actions, and feelings with beneficial thoughts, behaviors, and emotions. Addressing PE as a couple will help you develop new sexual and relationship meaning, a crucial resource in overcoming PE. Dealing with PE is an opportunity to deepen relationship intimacy by cooperating as an intimate team.

EXERCISE: SHARING YOUR FEELINGS ABOUT PE

Share with each other what PE has felt like and how it has affected you. When you learn to have good-enough sex, how do you want to feel then about sex? About each other?

Accepting the Complexity of PE

All of the features we have highlighted—physiology, cognitions, feelings, behaviors, and relationship identity, cooperation, and intimacy—intertwine as components of PE. Be aware of the complexity, but don't let it overwhelm you. Trust that you can address the important factors, and trust that your efforts will be good enough. By being so thorough, we offer you the opportunity to alleviate your distress and improve your sexual experience—to enjoy sex more and have great, intimate sex together!

4

Assessing Your PE

In this chapter, we will help you answer several important questions about your PE. How do you know if PE is really a problem? What are the criteria that differentiate PE from healthy sexual functioning? If you decide you do have PE, what kind or type of PE do you have? What are the causes? How severe is your PE? How do you decide what to do to resolve it? Will you need professional help?

When you determine the causes and severity of your PE, you take the most important step on the road to successfully resolving the problem. You know what you are dealing with and can set a course of action—individually and as a couple—to remedy your PE.

We will guide you through this process. You will need to be determined, patient, and decisive about using all your resources to help you to succeed. You may need to develop a more comfortable, cooperative relationship. You may need to find a wise and affirming physician for a medical evaluation. You may need to consult with a skilled and knowledgeable marital and sex therapist. Congratulate yourself for having the courage to face a difficult problem!

Do You Have PE?

We define PE as the inadvertent and unsatisfying rapid speed of male ejaculation. From a practical standpoint, you probably have PE if you are unable to decide or choose approximately when you want to ejaculate in more cases than not, and it is distressing to you and your partner. Consider the following four questions:

1. Can you choose when to ejaculate most of the time—in at least four out of five sexual experiences?

2. Are you able to relax well enough to enjoy sensuous physical pleasure during lovemaking? Is sex more than orgasm?

3. Are you able to relax and feel close and connected during lovemaking?

4. After you and your partner make love, are you both usually pleased and satisfied with your sexual experience?

If you are not able to answer yes to these questions, you are experiencing the common features of PE.

What Type of PE Do You Have?

To understand and remedy PE, it is crucial that you determine its cause or causes and develop a specific treatment plan. You learned about the nine causes of PE in chapter 3. We will help you examine each one so that you can take comprehensive, constructive action.

Diagnosing Your Type of PE

We will guide you through a step-by-step process to help you consider all of the causes that could be contributing to your PE. You want to be inclusive because if you miss a cause, you will overlook a potentially important factor in your change plan. Don't allow yourself to fail by an oversight. Be conservative. Assume any cause you suspect may be present until you know otherwise—that is, until you can rule it out as a factor.

Overview of PE Types

The PE diagnostic process leads you first through those types that are lifelong and then those that are acquired. Three types (neurologic system, psychological system, and psychosexual skills deficit) are considered when PE is lifelong, while six types (physical illness, physical injury, drug side-effect, psychological distress, relationship distress, and mixed) are considered when PE is acquired. The most common types of PE are neurologic system and psychosexual skills deficit. The next most common are relationship distress, psychological distress, and PE with another sexual dysfunction (usually erectile dysfunction). Occasionally we see physical illness PE (usually caused by prostate infection). It is rare to see psychological system PE, physical injury PE, or drug side-effect PE.

Your Personal Diagnostic Team

It is best to review the diagnostic decision-tree sequence with your partner so that you have a more comprehensive picture. Going through this together will be very useful later as you work as a team to resolve your PE.

It is wise to have a general physical examination with your family physician if you suspect a biological cause. Take the lead and ask your doctor to look for physical causes of your PE, especially focusing on identifying signs of general illness, chronic physical problems, localized genitourinary infection or inflammation, and signs of either generalized neurologic disease or localized sensory deficits that could cause or contribute to your PE.

EXERCISE: DIAGNOSING YOUR TYPE OF PE

As you follow these nine steps, note your answers on the PE Diagnostic Summary Sheet at the end of this chapter. Do not conclude that the first cause of PE is the only cause. Continue through each of the nine steps in order to determine all of the possible causes or manifestations.

Step 1: Do You Have Neurologic System PE?

Yes   No   Has PE occurred all your life?

Yes   No   Has PE occurred in all sexual situations (with different partners, during masturbation)?

Yes   No   Do you think that your penis has a physiological hypersensitivity; that is, does your penis feel supersensitive?

Yes   No   Does your ejaculation seem to be an unconscious reflex, an automatic reaction like an eye blink?

Yes   No   Are you confident that you do not have a serious, chronic psychological problem?

If you answered yes to most of these, you may have neurologic system PE.

Actually, it is not easy to conclusively diagnose neurologic system PE. There are several simple neurological examinations your physician or a neurologist may use, as well as some more involved tests like bulbocavernosus reflex (BCR) testing. Until you see a doctor, you usually will have to make an educated guess about the likelihood that you have neurologic system PE.

Step 2: Do You Have Psychological System PE?

Yes   No   Has PE occurred all your life?

Yes   No   Has PE occurred in all sexual situations?

Yes   No   Have you been diagnosed with—or do you think
you have—a chronic, psychological character
pattern or unrelenting problem such as obsessive-
compulsive disorder, chronic depression,
generalized anxiety disorder, or a personality
disorder such as dependent personality?

Yes   No   Have you taken a formal psychological test that
suggests you have a chronic psychological problem?

If you answered yes to the first two questions and at least one other, you may have psychological system PE.

While psychological system PE is rare, it is important to consider this because if you do not address the underlying cause, your efforts to remedy PE will be frustratingly unsuccessful. Careful evaluation will help sort out to what extent the psychological problem must be treated in order to resolve your PE.

Step 3: Do You Have Psychosexual Skills Deficit PE?

Yes   No   Has PE occurred all your life?

Yes   No   Has PE occurred in almost all situations, especially
with a partner?

Yes   No   Do you focus your sexual attention almost
exclusively on your partner—her body, actions, and
sexual responses?

Yes   No   Are you so mentally distracted that you are unable
to physically relax during sex or unable to focus on
the pleasure of your own bodily sensations of
arousal? If you have learned arousal pacing
strategies such as stop-start pacing, do you find
them difficult to use?

Yes   No   Are you unaware of your body's pelvic muscles
and how to use them for ejaculatory control?

Yes   No   Do you feel confused about your sexual response
and perplexed about how to regulate your sexual
arousal?

Yes   No   Do you feel shy about asking your partner for what
you want during sex?

Yes   No   Do you initiate and anxiously pursue sex with
              highly arousing activities such as oral sex or
              immediate intercourse rather than beginning slowly
              with relaxed kissing and light massaging?

If you answered yes to most of these, you may have psychosexual skills deficit PE.

Our program will be especially useful to you. We'll teach you
skills in managing your body during sexual arousal, regulating your
level of arousal, and cooperating with your partner.

Step 4: Do You Have Physical Illness PE?

Yes   No   Has your PE been acquired (developed after a
              period when you had adequate ejaculatory control
              and choice)?

Yes   No   Does your PE occur in all situations?

Yes   No   Has it been more than a year since you have had
              a general physical examination by your doctor
              which included a complete blood count and
              a prostate examination?

Yes   No   Do you have a family history of endocrine, blood,
              or neurologic irregularities (for example, multiple
              sclerosis)?

Yes   No   Did you or your partner contract a sexually
              transmitted disease recently?

Yes   No   Have you had, or do you have, a physical illness
              (such as prostatitis, neuritis, high blood pressure, or
              epilepsy) known to cause PE?

If you answered yes to the first two questions and at least one
other, you may have physical illness PE.

You will need thorough evaluation by a physician to determine
what condition might be causing or contributing to your PE. The
most common illnesses that cause PE are prostatitis (which can linger in a mild form for years without any obvious or clear symptoms
except for PE) and sexually transmitted diseases (for example,
chlamydia or gonorrhea).

Step 5: Do You Have Physical Injury PE?

Yes   No   Has your PE been acquired?

Yes   No   Does your PE occur in all situations?

Yes   No   Has there been a physical injury, spinal injury,
              pelvic surgery or trauma, or neurologic trauma that
              coincided with or was followed some time later
              by PE?

If you answered yes to all of these, you may have physical
injury PE.

If you suspect an injury may have caused your PE, consult with
your family physician, who will review your medical history and
recommend further testing.

Step 6: Do You Have Drug Side-Effect PE?

Yes   No   Has your PE been acquired?

Yes   No   Does your PE occur in all situations?

Yes   No   Have you recently stopped taking trifluoperazine
              (Novoflurazine, Solazine, Stelazine, Suprazine, or
              Terfluzine) or any opiate (for example, morphine)?

Yes   No   Are you taking a medication known to cause PE:
              Norpramin (desipramine), or a cold medication
              containing a form of ephedrine or pseudoephedrine
              (Sudafed, Actifed, Comtrex, Dristan, Sinutab,
              Robitussin, Triaminic, Broncholate, or Dimetane-DC)?

If you answered yes to the first two questions and at least one
other, you may have drug side-effect PE.

If you have recently discontinued one of the tranquilizers men-
tioned above or any opiate, PE is a common reaction. Allowing time
for the body to readjust usually clears up the PE. If the PE lasts more
than six to eight weeks, you should consider what else may be causing or maintaining your PE. If you suspect that your PE is caused by
a medication you're currently taking, talk with your doctor about
your medication dosage or options.

Step 7: Do You Have Psychological Distress PE?

Yes   No   Has your PE been acquired?

Yes   No   Does your PE occur in all situations?

Yes   No   Are you experiencing significant psychological
              distress such as depression, anxiety, grieving,
              career stress, or parenting problems? Have you
              recently gone through a major life transition such
              as a career change, moving your residence, the
              birth of your child, or sudden success?

Yes   No   Have you taken an objective psychological test that verifies you are experiencing psychological stress?

If you answered yes to the first two questions and at least one other, you may have psychological distress PE.

The critical difference between psychological system PE and psychological distress PE is its source and severity. Acquired psychological distress PE is a reaction to life events and is usually easier to treat.

Step 8: Do You Have Relationship Distress PE?

Yes   No   Has your PE been acquired?

Yes   No   Does PE occur only with your partner?

Yes   No   Has your partner recently expressed dissatisfaction with your general relationship?

Yes   No   Are you currently experiencing relationship distress such as poor communication, a deficit in emotional empathy, painful disagreements (fighting), or unresolved conflicts?

Yes   No   Have you recently taken an objective relationship test that suggests relationship distress?

Yes   No   Have you thought recently that marital or relationship therapy might be helpful?

If you answered yes to the first two questions and at least one other, you may have relationship distress PE.

Relationship distress PE is usually distinguished by acquired onset and situational occurrence in partner sex. In short, relationship deficiencies undermine the mutual emotional acceptance that is important to healthy sexual functioning.

Step 9: Do You Have PE with Another Sexual Dysfunction (Mixed PE)?

Yes   No   In addition to PE, do you experience another sexual problem such as erectile dysfunction, inhibited sexual desire, or pain in your penis during intercourse? Do you sometimes ejaculate without an erection?

Yes   No   Does this additional sexual dysfunction occur occasionally, frequently, or always?

If you answered yes to both of these, you may have PE with another sexual dysfunction (mixed PE).

It is normal to have sexual difficulties on occasion, but when this occurs regularly it represents a sexual dysfunction. Successful treatment of the other sexual problem can help resolve the PE.

How Severe Is Your PE?

Determining the severity of your PE will help you gain perspective on how challenging your PE is, how diligent you will need to be in addressing it, and the extent to which you could benefit from professional consultation. Take a moment to complete the Premature Ejaculation Severity Index (PESI). Make a copy and ask your partner to also complete the PESI. Although she will not know answers to some of the questions, her impressions of the severity of your PE can be very helpful.

EXERCISE: PREMATURE EJACULATION SEVERITY INDEX (PESI)

Circle the number that indicates what you typically experience for the questions below.

1. How long has premature or rapid ejaculation been a problem for you?

   10   9   8   7   6   5   4   3   2   1   0
   lifelong   intermittent   recent
                                (off and on)   or new
                                                              problem

2. In what percent of all sex acts are you unable to choose when to ejaculate?

   10   9   8   7   6   5   4   3   2   1   0
   100% 90% 80% 70% 60% 50% 40% 30% 20% 10% 0%

3. When do you usually ejaculate?

   10   9   8   7   6   5   4   3   2   1   0
   before   at   shortly   After
   penetration   penetration   after   some
                                        penetration   intercourse

4. If you can have intercourse, how long is it before you typically ejaculate?

10	9	8	7	6	5	4	3	2	1	0
not able to enter	15 sec	30 sec	1 min	2 min	3 min	4 min	5 min	10 min	15 min	more than 15 min

5. Rate the intensity or vigor of physical stimulation at the time of ejaculation.

10	9	8	7	6	5	4	3	2	1	0
very mild, little, or slow										very intense, vigorous, or fast

6. How difficult is it for you to control or choose when you ejaculate?

10	9	8	7	6	5	4	3	2	1	0
extremely difficult to control										extremely easy to control

7. How upset is your sexual partner by your premature ejaculation?

10	9	8	7	6	5	4	3	2	1	0
extremely troubled										very calm

8. How upset are you by your premature ejaculation?

10	9	8	7	6	5	4	3	2	1	0
extremely troubled										very calm

9. How much has your premature ejaculation affected your life in general?

10	9	8	7	6	5	4	3	2	1	0
major impact (for example, ruined relationship)										no significant effect

10. How often when you have sex do you also have desire or erection problems?

10	9	8	7	6	5	4	3	2	1	0
100%	90%	80%	70%	60%	50%	40%	30%	20%	10%	0%

Scoring the PESI

To determine your severity index, add your responses to items 1 through 10.

Total score: _____

Now enter your total score in the appropriate category below to indicate the severity of your PE.

_____ 0–20 Very mild severity

_____ 20–40 Mild severity

_____ 40–60 Moderate severity

_____ 60–80 High severity

_____ 80–100 Extreme severity

The lower your severity score, the more likely you are to be able to successfully resolve your PE. The more severe your PE is, the harder it will be to remedy and the more determined and disciplined you and your partner will need to be. If your case is of moderate severity, you have a good chance of addressing PE successfully through the techniques in this book, but you will need to invest a good amount of personal and relationship energy. If your PESI score indicates high or extreme severity, it will be difficult to resolve PE on your own, and it is very likely you would benefit from the coaching and support of a trained marital and sex therapist.

Summarizing What You Know about Your PE

At each step in the Diagnosing Your Type of PE exercise, you recorded your impression about what types of PE you may have on the PE Diagnostic Summary Sheet.

Now that you have completed the summary, review with your partner your findings on the causes or effects of your PE. What have you learned? What will you need to do to address PE together? What does your PESI score tell you about how difficult it will be to resolve your PE?

EXERCISE: PE DIAGNOSTIC SUMMARY SHEET

As you work through the diagnostic exercise in this chapter, mark the types of PE you think you may have. Where applicable, list the specific cause you suspect.

_____ Neurologic system PE

_____ Psychological system PE

(what condition? _____)

_____ Psychosexual skills deficit PE

_____ Physical illness PE

(what disease? _____)

_____ Physical injury PE

(what injury? _____)

_____ Drug side-effect PE

(what medication or drug? _____)

_____ Psychological distress PE

(what distress? _____)

_____ Relationship distress PE

(what distress? _____)

_____ PE with another sexual dysfunction (mixed PE)

(what other dysfunction? _____)

Your summary sheet offers you a comprehensive view of what areas you'll need to address in your action plan to resolve PE. If you think you may have a physiological or mixed type of PE, a medical checkup may help you confirm this. If you think you may have a psychological or mixed type of PE, a psychological consultation may help you confirm this.

In the following chapters, we will explain the different treatments and guide you to success. Treatments for physically based PE (neurologic system, physical illness, physical injury, or drug side-effect PE) are described in chapter 6. Treatments for psychologically based PE (psychological system, psychological distress, or relationship distress PE) are described in chapter 7. Treatments for psychosexual skills deficit PE—and for repairing individual and relationship damage from PE caused by other factors—is described in chapter 8. Mixed PE can be complicated and may require both physical and psychological treatments. If you are sure that your other sexual dysfunction (e.g., ED) is compensation for or overreaction to your PE, completing the exercises in the chapters that address the possible causes of your PE can be beneficial. Otherwise, consultation with your medical doctor and a professional marital and sex therapist is sensible.

Now that you've identified all the elements contributing to your PE, you can confidently engage in addressing these elements—and succeed!

5

Planning Your Treatment and Preparing for Action

Michael and Rebecca realized they would need to stay disciplined and focused if they were to master ejaculatory control. Michael had a number of factors causing and influencing his PE, and Rebecca's history of childhood sexual abuse and disappointing relationships made her sexual desire fragile. Fortunately, both were motivated to make sexuality a positive component of their marital bond.

Michael and Rebecca were successful in learning ejaculatory control because they understood the importance of integrating the cognitive, behavioral, emotional, and interpersonal dimensions of sexuality. It was crucial for Michael and Rebecca to adopt positive sexual attitudes. Michael was strongly influenced by traditional male socialization, believing that if he "failed" at intercourse, he was a failure as a man. Michael actually had high sexual desire but felt so humiliated by PE that he avoided sex with Rebecca. Instead, Michael compulsively masturbated, which caused him to feel guilty and Rebecca to feel rejected. Gradually, Michael and Rebecca learned to acknowledge the positive functions of sexuality. Especially important for Rebecca was to accept that the essence of sexuality is giving and receiving pleasure-oriented touching. This was totally different than her childhood experiences with abusive sexuality.

Michael focused on learning the sensual self-entrancement and arousal pacing techniques during partner sex (we'll teach these in chapter 8). Together, they adopted an antiavoidance approach. Michael realized that to learn ejaculatory control, he needed to act, not agonize or apologize.

Michael and Rebecca developed a warm sexuality which was mutual, pleasurable, and intimate. Michael viewed Rebecca as his intimate sexual friend and ally in learning ejaculatory control. With time, they achieved the fundamental aim of ejaculatory control: increasing their individual sexual pleasure, increasing each other's pleasure, and enhancing their relationship by prolonging and enjoying sexual arousal. They focused not on perfect sexual performance but on sharing sexual pleasure.

In this chapter, we'll help you follow a similar path to success. You will work with your partner to develop a treatment plan for your PE. You will learn how to prepare yourself and your relationship—cognitively, behaviorally, and emotionally—for healing from PE. To help you think differently about PE, we'll discuss the multiple purposes of sex, the three basic types of sexual arousal, and their relevance to learning ejaculatory control.

Developing Your Treatment Plan

Based on the causes and severity of your PE, which you determined in chapter 4, you now can decide on strategies to change it. Chapters 6, 7, and 8 will help you through the steps to take in each of the major areas: physiological, psychological, and relational. This section will help you decide where to focus your efforts.

Strategies for Physically Caused PE

If you indicated the possibility of physically caused PE (neurologic system PE, physical illness PE, physical injury PE, or drug side-effect PE), focus on the strategies in chapter 6. If you think you may have a physiological or mixed type of PE, a medical checkup may help you confirm your type.

Strategies for Psychological and Relational PE

If you indicated the possibility of psychological system PE, psychological distress PE, or relationship distress PE, carefully read chapter 7. If you think you may have a psychological or mixed type of PE, a psychological evaluation may help confirm your type and develop a treatment strategy. There are some additional self-help steps you may want to consider.

- Consult a well-respected book about the type of distress you suspect.

- Seek feedback from your partner or someone else you trust.

- If you suspect psychological system PE, consider what you know about your family history (for example, "Grandpa was always depressed").

- Search for psychology information and self-tests at trustworthy Internet sites (see the Resources section).

Strategies for Psychosexual Skills Deficit PE

If you indicated the possibility of psychosexual skills deficit PE, focus on chapter 8.

Strategies for Coping with the Detrimental Effects of PE

Regardless of the cause of your PE, the strategies in chapters 7, 8, 9, and 10 can help you heal the detrimental effects of PE on your well-being and the well-being of your relationship.

Preparing Yourself for the Work Ahead

Unless you have a simple, biologically caused type of PE that can be solved with direct medical treatment, you will need to learn new skills. The skills have cognitive, behavioral, emotional, and relational components. They are designed to help you affirm yourself, relax your body, focus on your physical sensations, increase your pleasure, and deepen your relationship closeness as well as control ejaculation. Your efforts, step-by-step, will pay off with wonderful feelings of satisfaction with yourself, your partner, and your lovemaking. Yes, these skills are an effort; there is no easy fix. But it will be worth it.

Here are the key points to remember:

- You have to pursue *all* of the dimensions of your PE.

- Remember that you are a complete person with thoughts, feelings, and behaviors.

- Satisfying sex is a skill like any other physical or emotional activity you have come to enjoy.

- As you approach learning the skills to manage PE, keep your "relationship" perspective. Don't lose sight of the big picture.

- Understand clearly your objectives: keep in mind what you are trying to learn at each step.

- Patiently practice the specific skills for success and cooperate with your partner.

- Closeness and satisfaction is the ultimate goal.

Is Sex a Skill?

One of the common myths about sex is that it is supposed to be "natural" or automatic, like eating and sleeping. Reproductive sex does appear to be biologically natural. But the other functions of sex—heightened pleasure, personal self-esteem, and relationship intimacy—are achieved by learning psychosexual skills.

Think of any skill that brings satisfaction, especially a physical activity: dancing, skiing, swimming, climbing, hang gliding, parachuting, even running. Marathon runners don't just go out and do it. It takes discipline, concentration, psychological preparation, physical conditioning, and learning pacing strategies. So if you want to become a "marathoner" during sex, you'll need some mental and physical preparation—some "training." Yes, biological sex is basically natural—penis goes into vagina—but to really enjoy emotionally intimate sex takes attention, knowledge, and practice. Yes, it is annoying to have to give such careful attention to something you wish would just "flow." But if you have PE, managing arousal takes training. That is a fact.

A skill, whether cognitive, emotional, behavioral, or interpersonal, is the learned ability to perform the task well and with some ease. Skills are developed through practice (repetition), persistence (discipline), and patience. Can you remember learning new skills as a child? Learning to ride a bike, for example, required a certain degree of persistence and self-regulation of the fear of falling down. You had to try time after time until it became "natural." You probably tipped over, skinned a knee now and then, but didn't give up. Managing PE means using practice, persistence, and patience to learn cognitive, emotional, behavioral, and relational skills.

Cognitive Preparation

The most important sex organ in your body is between your ears: your mind. During the skills training, you will want to be a kind but strong "gatekeeper," noticing what you are thinking and where your attention is focused. Negative, pessimistic, self-defeating, or distracting thoughts will not help. By focusing on the opportunity of each step and exercise, you will do well. It is essential that you learn to focus your attention and discipline your mind.

If you think that the training in this book will be too difficult, reassure yourself that these skills are very manageable because you do them in increments, not all at once. Accept that you might not feel optimistic now; after all, you have tried so hard for so long without real success. It is understandable that you fear that our comprehensive approach might not work. That's fine. The details may look foreboding, but optimism is the caboose on the train. Wait for it. But in the meantime, prepare yourself mentally to relax and engage in the process.

Have a Positive Attitude toward Sex and a Deep Commitment to Mutual Sexual Health

The first step is to consciously affirm the positive value of healthy, physical, bodily sexuality. Sex is good. Pleasure is good. You do not have to numb pleasure to learn ejaculatory control.

Take Personal Responsibility for Pursuing Sexual Growth

Take personal responsibility for your sexual responsiveness. Be sexually responsible for yourself—be accountable. There are individual skills that the man is responsible for learning, skills his partner is responsible for learning, and skills the couple learns cooperatively. Some of the more effective skills are neither commonsense nor attainable without diligent effort. Being responsible means intentionally engaging in the change steps.

Prepare Yourself to Relax

The treatment steps will help you work through stresses that undermine the physiological relaxation essential to healthy sexuality. Realistic expectations based on accurate knowledge of sexual functioning are reassuring; they are the cognitive precursors of physiological relaxation.

Understanding the multiple purposes of sex can help you maintain realistic expectations and contribute to your and your partner's motivation to be flexible, patient, and cooperative.

The Four Purposes of Sex

Why do you have sex? If you are not sure why you are having sex, you are more likely to have a problem. Automatic sex may procreate, but it commonly falls short in the intimacy department.

Sexual science suggests that there are four purposes or functions for sex.

Reproduction. Procreation is the "natural" or biological function of sex.

Physical pleasure. Sensual enjoyment and physical pleasure is a basic function of sex, especially in long-term, satisfying sexual relationships.

Self-esteem. Individuals seek enhancement of their psychological self-esteem through sex and pursue feelings of self-worth, confidence, and pride in being a sexual person.

Relationship benefits. The interpersonal function of sex is to foster love, intimacy, affection, joy, closeness, and couple satisfaction.

In healthy relationships, sex has multiple positive purposes. In dysfunctional relationships, the purposes are distorted or negative: manipulation, destructive control, or hurt. Yet even in healthy relationships, a single reason for sex can eclipse all the others—for instance, during infertility protocols when sex must occur at a particular time and under particular circumstances—and the pressures of one-dimensional sex undermine other benefits like pleasure and intimacy and can cause PE, erectile dysfunction, or inhibited sexual desire.

PE and the Purposes of Sex

PE interferes with the positive functions of sex, bringing distress to both the man and his partner. PE becomes intensely stressful for the man as he becomes preoccupied with pleasing his partner, trying to delay ejaculation in order to prevent the frustration and hurt of a disrupted sexual experience. While he may be able to impregnate, he finds very limited sensual or physical pleasure in sex, suffers a loss of self-esteem, and feels tremendous shame and frustration about being the source of hurt and damage in their intimate relationship. His partner experiences frustration with each of the purposes of sex as well: a diminution of physical pleasure, loss of self-esteem, and confusing feelings of relational hurt and abandonment. As long as the man is focused solely on performance and thus experiences the outcome of sex to be negative, he will suffer performance anxiety that exacerbates and reinforces PE. If you are to resolve PE, you must think about sex in terms of pleasure, self-esteem, and intimacy as well as good-enough ejaculatory control.

The Styles of Sexual Arousal

Learning that your partner may have different reasons for having sex and different ways of getting aroused helps couples appreciate and accept their differences. It also helps you feel respect and acceptance from the other as you mutually pursue satisfying sex. This is an important aspect of how you think about sex.

In our experience, men with PE invariably and exclusively use arousal strategies where the focus of erotic attention is on the partner. To try to slow ejaculation, they use "spectatoring" (detached self-observation) or other distraction techniques. This diverts your focus from your own body and your own sensual experience, and subsequently diminishes your ability to manage your sexual arousal. In addition, men with PE initiate and pursue sex with highly arousing activity (we call this sexual drag racing), rather than beginning calmly and then gradually increasing stimulation. You may fail to connect with your sensuality or even try to dissociate from physical sensations during sexual activity. You may find it difficult to enjoy the physical sensations in your whole body during arousal.

Let's take a look at the range of sexual arousal styles. We have adapted Mosher's (1980) suggestions and distinguished three basic styles of arousal.

Sensual self-entrancement occurs through focusing on your own physical sensations and sensual pleasure. Your attention is focused primarily on your own body.

Partner interaction occurs through focusing on your partner: her body, her responses, and the "sexy" or "romantic" interaction with her. Your attention is outside your body.

Role enactment occurs through your private imagination or fantasy, role-playing with your partner, or acting out feelings or fantasies. Your attention is outside your body and more broadly focused than in partner interaction arousal.

These styles are differentiated by where you focus your attention. Each style leads to a particular kind of behavior. For example, the person who pursues arousal by partner interaction is active, eyes open, focused on the interaction, looking at the partner, talkative (engaging in romantic or "sweet" talk), and energetic. This is the sexual style commonly portrayed on television and in movies—passionate and impulsive. The person is turned on by focusing attention outside himself, enjoying the partner, and getting carried away in passion and eroticism.

On the other hand, the individual pursuing arousal primarily by sensual self-entrancement immerses in his sensory experience and closes his eyes, goes within, becomes quiet, and may look detached and passive. Routine, sameness, and stylized touch help him to get turned on.

The person aroused by role enactment enjoys sexual variety and experimentation such as the partner dressing in sexy lingerie, role-playing being "tough" or "hard to get," acting out a scene from a movie or fantasy, having sex in new places like at a hotel or outdoors, or using "toys" like massage oil or a vibrator or dildo. By trying new things, the person finds excitement and arousal through sexual playfulness, freedom, and uniqueness. As with partner inter-action arousal, the focus is on scenarios outside your body.

While individuals usually have a preference for one style, every person has the capacity for arousal by each style and may use them interchangeably. For example, you may begin lovemaking with play-ful teasing (role enactment), change to enjoying touching your part-ner and seeing her naked body (partner interaction), and then switch to focusing on the sensations you feel in your own body while being touched (entrancement). Your use of the three styles can vary over time. Individuals and couples may go through developmental stages. For example, early in a couple's sexual life, partner interaction arousal is common, giving way to sensual self-entrancement arousal and a more sedate sexuality, then enlivened with role enactment or a resurgence of partner interaction arousal. This process can explain why couples who have mild cases of PE early in their relationship "grow out of it" with relaxation and routine induced by familiarity. Some couples pursue a different type of arousal from one sexual meeting to the next: Tuesday, self-entrancement "because I was tired"; Saturday, partner interaction arousal "because I was really turned on by my partner."

Understanding the Styles for Acceptance and Flexibility

Sexual partners who do not realize that there are different kinds of arousal may misinterpret their partner's behavior as hurtful and take it personally. For example, the primarily self-entrancement-focused woman having sex with a man aroused by partner interaction finds his lovemaking efforts (the looking, talking, heavy breathing, interacting, being expressive and passionate) distracting and wonders why he is disturbing her focus and working against her arousal. This man, on the other hand, might interpret his lover's self-entrancement style—quiet and inward-focused—as disinterested, aloof, bored, or even rejecting. The potential for misunderstanding and hurt is evident.

You need to understand your partner's sexual arousal style to interpret each other's behavior correctly. This illustrates the importance of sharing your sexual feelings, cooperating, and collaborating in pleasure. This mutual understanding is crucial to your success in the work ahead.

Be a Skeptic at First

What if you doubt that you can overcome PE? It's okay to have a hesitant or doubtful attitude. This is not to encourage you to be pessimistic, but rather to remind you that you can't force the change you seek. You probably have already tried this, and it has failed you. You don't have to believe in the skills to benefit from them. So it's fine to be a doubting Thomas or an honorary Missourian, adopting the state motto: Show me. You do not have to make the skills work; let the skills show you the way. All you have to do is relax and focus. Just show up, so to speak, and do each step well enough.

Here are the key points to remember as you prepare yourself mentally:

- Learn a positive attitude toward your body, sex, and lovemaking, with a conscious commitment to mutual sexual satisfaction.

- Take responsibility for your improvement.

- Operate from accurate knowledge and realistic expectations of lovemaking.

- Realize that there are multiple purposes for sex. Don't be trapped in a rigid performance focus.

- Be aware of the styles of arousal.

- Be a skeptic! Free yourself by adopting a show-me attitude toward the steps.

- Remember that what and how you think directly influences how you feel and what you do.

Emotional Preparation

You probably feel burdened by your PE, but you can begin to let that feeling subside. You are a complete person, and by restructuring the way you think about yourself as a sexual person and learning to change how you function, you will come to feel better about yourself and your partner. The way you think and what you do influences how you feel.

Accept Your Honest Feelings about PE

Prepare yourself for the steps ahead by accepting that you may have felt any of a long list of detrimental feelings: discouragement, hurt, frustration, humiliation, anger, confusion, apprehension, embarrassment, shame, guilt, depression, anxiety, worry, sadness, bitterness. These feelings are reminding you that you are not satisfied with the way things are. It is time to change. Help prepare yourself for change by accepting these negative feelings. Acceptance of your honest emotional experience is an essential preparation for growth. Having feelings does not mean you must act on them or feel controlled by them. Our change program will help create a comfort zone or safe harbor where the emotional hurts are manageable.

During the learning experiences in the steps ahead, be sure to focus on your physical sensations. The sensual self-entrancement arousal training, in particular, will help you accept and calm your feelings. By focusing on your sensations, you will help yourself to stop worrying about PE and feeling bad about sex. Calm, conscientious focus on your own sensations will become your ally.

Distinguish Your Feelings from Your Behaviors

Make the distinction between being aware of your emotions (feeling) and expressing your emotions (behavior). Recognize the importance of owning your emotions, but realize there are risks and harm in expressing unbridled negative feelings. Certainly do not express destructive feelings as you work on the exercises together. Internally soothe your negative feelings and remember that you can choose to develop positive feelings through new behaviors. Expressing negative feelings will only trap you in the past, and this will be very discouraging for you both. If it seems impossible to manage your feelings, this is an indication that you and your partner could benefit from marital or sex therapy.

Here are the key points to remember as you prepare yourself emotionally:

- Your feelings are important. Your sexual feelings are a big part of the glue that holds your relationship together. Feelings flow from how you are thinking and what you are doing.

- Don't let old negative feelings run your life. Accept those feelings, but don't let them interfere with new learning and behaviors.

- Focus on your physical sensations to stop your mind from worrying about PE.

- Do not express unbridled anger, frustration, or resentment during your sexual work together. Acknowledge and internally calm these emotions and give yourself a chance to grow.

Behavioral Preparation

Prepare yourself for the behavioral tasks by reminding yourself of the need for self-discipline: regulation of your thoughts, feelings, behaviors, and interactions. Yes, it is a bummer that you have to work at this, but good things are built by effort. It is a good idea to schedule your practice of the steps. Set aside the time and make each step a priority. It will be hard at times, but it is necessary. Suck it up!

Be sure to consider the environment in which you'll be doing your skills learning. Many use the privacy of the bedroom, although any secure, private, comfortable place is fine. Make sure it is free from interruptions, since the goal is to create a safe place for relaxation and undivided attention and focus.

Cultivate Self-Discipline

Doing the steps requires disciplined concentration on the pleasure in your body, a steady and dedicated commitment and determination to do the exercises day in, day out, over a number of weeks to develop your skills.

Dedicate Yourself to Physical Relaxation

Learning detailed, physiologically focused relaxation techniques is essential to ejaculatory control. It is counterintuitive, but the body performs better when relaxed. Most men (and women) just cannot believe that relaxation is essential for good sexual functioning. It is not common sense. You can take our word for it, or you can think about this: Medications like Viagra help many men who have erectile dysfunction, including men who also have PE. How does Viagra work? Technically, this pill facilitates a chemical process unique to enzymes in the penis that ultimately relaxes the muscles surrounding the microscopic arteries, which in turn dilates the arteries causing blood to engorge the penis, and voilà: an erection! The point is that even artificially induced relaxation brings about an erection.

The mechanism for ejaculation is not a direct one, but rather a psychological one. Men who ejaculate quickly because they worry about maintaining a sufficient erection, when reassured by Viagra, are thought to relax more, to not watch themselves so anxiously, and because of the general relaxation, also last longer. Think about it, men: Physiological relaxation helps sexual functioning.

Do the Steps in Order

The skills development exercises in chapters 7 and 8 should be followed in order. Working ahead or skipping steps would be like jumping into a swimming pool before you know how to swim! We know you want to get to the good stuff. But patience is your friend. Moving too quickly will undermine your ability to relax, which is essential to progress. Take one step at a time, one exercise at a time, one stage at a time. Remember the Chinese proverb, A journey of one thousand miles begins with a single step.

Just Be Good Enough

It is essential that you understand what you are trying to do and that you train yourself sufficiently to bring about changes in the way you make love. The painful reality is that the way you have been approaching sex has not worked. This means you must work hard enough to bring about change, but you only need to learn and do the skills well enough. Do not pressure yourself to be perfect. In fact, it is important that you do not work too hard, because to succeed, you must relax your mind and body. Striving for perfection produces performance pressure and undermines your relaxation. So we encourage you to practice the principle of just being good enough.

Learn Sensual Self-Entrancement Arousal

Learning to trust sexual arousal by focusing on sensations in your own body is essential to ejaculatory control. Men usually don't believe this is possible, let alone normal. You will find erections effortless and ejaculatory control easier when you learn to base your arousal in sensual self-entrancement. During the skills work in chapter 8, you will recognize that self-entrancement arousal is built into the steps and encourages you to relax physically while sexually aroused. You will truly find this arousal remarkable when you begin to integrate it with the other steps to ejaculatory control and building intimacy.

Here are some key points to remember about behavior:

- Realize you must discipline yourself—regulate your thoughts, feelings, and actions. Yes, it is difficult.

- Learn to physically relax during arousal. It is an essential skill.

- Do the steps in the proper sequence.

- Do not push to be perfect. Just be good enough!

- Learn sensual self-entrancement sexual arousal.

Interpersonal Preparation

You want to "fix" your penis and your ejaculation speed, yet remember that the most important goal and predictor of success—and the greatest reward—is your relationship intimacy. If you are working within a self-defeating environment, you will not succeed. On the other hand, if you have addressed the relationship hurt and divisiveness that have resulted from the PE and found relationship forgiveness and healing, your intimate relationship will help you to succeed at PE management. Your relationship is the "system" or environment for your sexual growth. Be careful not to overlook the essential importance of mutual support and acceptance. Keep your perspective. Remember that your PE is but one aspect of your overall relationship.

Sexual Cooperation Is Essential

While you can learn the skills for slowing ejaculation on your own, it works best to do so with your lover so your intimate relationship is working cooperatively. Cooperation provides a safe environment for learning the skills and gives both partners the opportunity to heal from the old anguish. The process itself invites cooperation and closeness.

Putting the other person first builds resentments when it is not reciprocated. When both put the other's feelings and happiness first, the emotional benefits can be wonderful. We call this the "give to get" pleasuring principle.

Prioritize Mutual Emotional Empathy

Emotional empathy (acceptance, affirmation, comfort, support, understanding) is the glue of intimacy. It is fundamentally important in healthy, satisfying relationships. Above all else, most individuals look to their marriage for empathy and emotional comfort.

Forgive Yourself and Your Partner

Forgive yourself and your partner for the hurt and disappointment—no matter how small or how monumental—that you've experienced around sexuality. This requires a commitment. If you do not forgive, your emotions will block your ability to focus on your body's sensations, to relax your body, and to learn the skills. What is the shortcut to forgiveness? Be aware that the hurt was in the past. The future can feel different. And with your partner? Say you are sorry and ask for forgiveness and acceptance now.

Here are the key points to remember as you prepare your relationship for the changes ahead:

- Relationship intimacy is your ultimate goal and your ultimate reward.

- Relationship cooperation is essential.

- Verbally forgive yourself and your partner for the past sexual hurt, pain, conflict, disappointment, and alienation. Do not hold yourself and each other emotionally hostage for the past.

- Talk with your partner about your sexual feelings. This will help generate mutual understanding, empathy, and acceptance. This will also help you develop personal comfort with sex and learn more about your partner.

- Keep your perspective. Satisfying sex is rooted in a healthy relationship.

You may be feeling overwhelmed by the task ahead. Remember that change is a process, and be willing to learn as you go. By preparing yourself cognitively, emotionally, behaviorally, and interpersonally, you give yourself the best possible chance to succeed in managing PE. Be calm. Be patient. Be open. Don't worry about being perfect. Just be good enough!

6

Medical, Pharmacologic, and Physiological Treatments

PE that originates from a biological cause needs treatment that addresses the physiological problem. In this chapter we will discuss the medical treatments and options for the four kinds of PE with physical or biological causes. If these problems are a primary factor in your PE, you need to carefully consider medical and physiological interventions, or you will face disappointment and frustration in your attempt to develop ejaculatory control. Remember, you want to address all the factors involved in your type of PE and to use all your resources—including medical treatment, medication, and physiological aids—to learn ejaculatory control.

Addressing the Medical Side of PE

In this chapter you will learn how to determine if you need a medical evaluation and how to work comfortably with your physician. Then we will describe the treatments for the biological types of PE: neurologic system PE, physical illness PE, physical injury PE, and drug side-effect PE. There are a number of medications that have the effect of slowing PE, as well as several other medical options for managing PE. It is important to consider how to integrate these medical interventions into your couple sexual relationship.

How to Determine Whether You Need a Medical Evaluation

If you noted the possibility of a physical type of PE on your PE Diagnostic Summary Sheet in chapter 4, it is important that you discuss the problem with your physician. Your doctor can not only determine whether your PE could have a physical cause but also offer a medical or pharmacological treatment. For example, if you confirm that you have lifelong neurologic system PE, your doctor can help you consider in detail the use of medications. Or, if your PE is acquired, your doctor can examine your prostate to see whether an infection has caused PE. Your physician could also be your best professional case manager, referring you to other trustworthy physicians who specialize in sexual medicine, as well as psychologists, marital therapists, or sex therapists.

How to Work Comfortably with Your Physician

Talking about your sexual concerns is likely something you are not very comfortable doing. People talk about sex in general, but few discuss their own sexuality, especially sexual difficulties. It is hard for many to believe that nearly 50 percent of adults have sex problems, sexual dysfunction, or sexual dissatisfaction (Laumann, Paik, and Rosen 1999). Physicians and other health professionals in general medical practice rarely recognize existing sexual problems or dysfunctions in their patients.

Do not fault your doctor, because he or she lives in the same society with the same discomforts. Most physicians assume that if sexual concerns are important to you as the patient, you will initiate discussion about it, while at the same time you may assume that since your doctor has the professional training and the ability to help with sexual problems, he or she will lead the inquiry and discussion. Unfortunately, these attitudes serve to continue a silent avoidance of sexual concerns, leaving you to worry privately without receiving help.

We suggest that you take the lead, because your physician may not. By raising the subject, you gain a sense of control over the process. Your leadership can provide focus.

How to Talk with Your Doctor

Use your own impressions to determine whether your doctor is likely to be comfortable talking about sexual concerns. Don't be distressed if he or she seems uncomfortable at first, because most physicians have received very little specific training in sexual medicine. Most doctors very much want to be helpful and will be willing to sort out the medical aspects with you.

Here are some suggestions for starting the discussion:

I want to talk to you about a sexual concern I have, but I am embarrassed.

I'm having a sex problem that I'd like your help with.

I would like to ask you about a sex problem that I'm having. Do you think you can help me?

Can you refer me to a sexual medicine specialist?

My impression is that you don't specialize in sexual concerns, but can you refer me to a doctor who does?

Depending on your suspicions about what is causing your PE, you might ask your doctor a specific question:

For the past six months, I've noticed that I ejaculate quickly, and I wonder if I might have a physical illness that is causing this.

I wonder if I have a prostate infection. Should I have an exam, or should we do some testing?

I'm reading a book about premature ejaculation, and it suggests that since it's been a problem for over a year, I should talk to you to make sure I don't have a prostate infection or some other illness that could cause PE.

You can even take this book along to show your doctor the section in chapter 4 where we list some of the illnesses that can cause PE.

Your doctor does not have to be comfortable talking with patients about sex to be a really good doctor; it just helps a lot. Your doctor may be waiting for you to ask. Give him or her a chance to help you.

Thank your doctor for being willing to talk with you about your sexual concerns or offering you a referral. Then, as you leave the office, congratulate yourself for taking the lead and being your own sexual health advocate.

What's Involved in a Medical Evaluation

Your general physician (whether an internist or family practi-tioner), who knows you and your medical history best, is the likely first choice to discuss your concerns about PE. You may be referred to an urologist or sexual medicine specialist for further evaluation. Medical evaluation for PE typically consists of three steps.

History

Your doctor will talk with you about your experience of PE. This discussion may include general background, some basic information about when and how fast you ejaculate, your personal medical history, a brief sexual history, other symptoms or aspects of your medical situation, your ideas of the cause, and how distressed you are. Your doctor is trying to gain a more comprehensive understanding of your situation as well as rule out some medical possibilities that could cause your sexual problem.

Physical Examination

Your doctor will examine your body, focusing on your genital area, and will check your prostate gland for signs of infection.

Testing

Some blood and urine tests may also be done to make sure there is no systemic problem. If your doctor suspects a prostate infection, he or she may want to take a sample of the fluid in the prostate to determine the kind of infection.

Treatments for Neurologic System PE

By far the most common physiological type of PE is caused by an overly efficient neurological system. In other words, your ejaculatory reflex is hardwired to go off quickly.

If you think you have neurologic system PE, there are a number of options for you to consider. Because neurologic system PE is hard-wired in your body and that hardwiring cannot be overhauled, we recommend that you try the psychosexual skills program in chapter 8 first to try to compensate for your overly efficient neurologic system. If your case is particularly severe (you have a PESI score above 80 or you often ejaculate before you can enter your partner's vagina), then the most promising medical treatment is medication that acts on the nervous system to slow ejaculation.

There are international reports (Tullii, Guillaux, et al. 1994; Schapiro 1943) that surgery (severing nerves in the penis to deaden sensation or destroying tissue in the prostate) can slow rapid ejaculation. The fact that some men resort to permanent injury to their bodies to try to resolve PE demonstrates how profoundly distressing PE can feel. We consider these treatments inappropriate and unethical because they are not only intrusive, radical, and unnecessary, but also irreversible. In addition, we have found that particularly detailed training in the psychosexual skills we'll teach in chapter 8, combined with medication, is helpful for the great majority of men. We also want to remind you to understand PE in the larger perspective of intimacy and relationship cooperation. If you have neurologic system PE that is not severe, accepting the biological reality and cooperatively adapting to it may be the most positive resolution.

Pharmacologic Interventions

A variety of antidepressants or antianxiety medications may neurologically slow down ejaculation, allowing some men to last two to ten times as long. The benefit may not be profound—for the man who ejaculates in ten to fifteen seconds, lasting ten times as long may mean only two minutes of intercourse—but for the man with chronic and severe PE, this may be quite satisfying. We recommend that you consider medication if your PE is exceptionally severe, if it doesn't respond to the psychosexual skills approach, or in conjunction with sex therapy. Some medications are taken daily, while others are taken several hours before sex.

Using medication is not a sign of weakness but a choice, and many men find it an important resource in gaining ejaculatory control. However, for some men, medication use implies the need to depend on an external resource rather than their own ability and does not support sexual self-esteem. Pharmacologic treatment alone is often insufficient because of the lack of effect in some men, the reluctance of some men to consistently use prescription medications, or complicating psychological and relationship factors. There are also concerns about the unknown effects of long-term use of medications for PE management.

Medication must be prescribed and monitored by a physician. Weighing the costs and the benefits of using medications is part of your decision making as a couple. For some men, obtaining the desired effect of inhibiting ejaculation can be a matter of trial and error of different medications and dosages. New medical treatments for PE are being developed. Ask your doctor what is currently available. We strongly advise against self-medication with alcohol, recreational drugs, or some over-the-counter remedies, as they have their own obvious risks.

Antidepressants

The *selective serotonin reuptake inhibitor* (SSRI) antidepressants Prozac (fluoxetine), Zoloft (sertraline), Paxil (paroxetine), Luvox (fluvoxamine), and Effexor (venlafaxine) are increasingly used to aid men who suffer PE, capitalizing on a common side-effect of inhibiting ejaculation. Studies and clinical experience confirm that these medications delay ejaculation in 20 to 60 percent of cases. These drugs increase the level of serotonin, and higher serotonin levels are thought to inhibit ejaculation. These medications are taken daily.

An older class of antidepressants known as *tricyclics*, including Anafranil (clomipramine) and Elavil (amitriptyline), also commonly delay ejaculation. These medications increase levels of both serotonin and norepinephrine. Anafranil has been frequently studied and is noted to be very effective in inhibiting ejaculation when taken two to four hours before the desired effect, especially for men who are prone to be "spectators" in the bedroom and are highly anxious about PE. The tricyclics, however, have more inconvenient side effects than the SSRIs (for example, dry mouth).

Antianxiety Medications

Antianxiety medicines, if properly prescribed, may also be useful. A number of medications that are effective in treating generalized anxiety and panic attacks can help some men slow down ejaculation. These medications include Librium (chlordiazepoxide), Ativan (lorazepam), Valium (diazepam), and Xanax (alprazolam). However, the inhibiting effect of these medications on ejaculation is limited and not as dramatic as the effect of SSRIs, and they help less than 10 percent of men with PE. These medications are taken one to four hours before beginning sex.

Anesthetic Creams

Numbing creams have long been used to slow ejaculation by deadening the sensations in the penis. If you use these creams, you must then use a condom so that the cream does not numb your partner's vagina as well. There are, for convenience, condoms (Detane, Mandelay, Performax) that you can buy over the counter with an anesthetic (benzocaine) already packaged inside.

We understand some men feel desperate to slow ejaculation and believe that they need to use anesthetics. We believe this is unnecessary and an ill-advised quick fix that does not really solve the issues of PE and cooperative lovemaking. To deaden the pleasure in your penis is contrary to our approach, which is designed to increase your pleasure, enhance intimacy with your partner, and teach you to saturate your body with pleasure while you maintain ejaculatory control.

Combination Treatments

Some physicians experiment with combination treatments that include a number of medications designed to overwhelm the neurologic system and reduce psychological anxiety. In severe cases of PE, multiple treatments may be effective. For example, Viagra may be used to ensure erection and overcome the fear of erectile dysfunction, while an anesthetic cream may be applied to numb the penis and an antidepressant medication may be used to calm and inhibit ejaculation.

Devices for Premature Ejaculation

In addition to pharmacologic treatments, devices are sometimes used, although they have not been scientifically proven to be effective.

Testicular Restraint Device

Some men have found that they can slow ejaculation by cuffing the testicles in the hand and gently pulling or holding down. Although not approved for use by the U.S. Food and Drug Administration, Velcro-type devices that restrain testicular ascent are available through mail order (often advertised in erotic magazines) and drugstores.

Penile Rubber Ring Device

British psychiatrists Wise and Watson (2002) have reported a small pilot study that used a latex rubber ring on the base of the penis daily for no more than thirty minutes, but not during sex. Some of the men reported that they improved ejaculatory control within a week of using the device. It may be that the device desensitized or stressed the penile nerves or operated as a *placebo* (that is, it worked simply because the men expected it to).

Biofeedback Training

Rome urologists La Pera and Nicastro (1996) devised an extensive pelvic muscle training program similar to that used in treating incontinence. This method includes three techniques—pelvic muscle exercises, electrostimulation, and biofeedback—taught in twenty sessions, three times per week. The training strengthens the pelvic muscles and teaches men to recognize and control contraction of these muscles. Approximately 60 percent of men with PE are helped by this technique. La Pera and Nicastro's work reinforces the importance of the pelvic muscles in ejaculatory control.

Treatments for Physical Illness PE

Your physician can treat medical disorders that directly cause PE. Inflammatory disorders such as infection of the prostate or urethra are treated with antibiotics that target the particular organism causing the infection.

Evaluation for diabetes and over- or underactivity of the thyroid gland may be necessary if the history and physical examination suggest a problem with these endocrine systems.

Treatments for Physical Injury PE

Medical treatments for the specific injuries that cause PE (such as spinal cord injury, head injury, trauma to the sympathetic nervous system, pelvic fractures and other torso traumas, or localized sensory impairment) are currently very limited. When such injury results in permanent physiological damage, treatment with medications that slow ejaculation may offer help for some. Sex therapy can help you learn to adapt to a permanent impairment. Chapters 8 and 9 offer some guidance here.

Treatments for Drug Side-Effect PE

Because this type of PE is caused by either withdrawal from or use of specific drugs, treatment is generally straightforward. When PE is caused by drug withdrawal, normal sexual functioning will return after the chemical leaves the body and the body rebalances. This may require from two to six weeks, depending on the medication. When PE results from a medication you are taking, you and your doctor should discuss the possibility of stopping or switching to a different medication if it is safe to do so. If normal function does not return, you should suspect additional or other causes of your PE.

Treatments for PE with Another Sexual Dysfunction (Mixed PE)

A medical examination can help identify physical causes for each sexual dysfunction—erectile dysfunction or inhibited desire—in addition to the PE. Specialized tests such as duplex ultrasound, cavernosometry or cavernosography, nocturnal penile tumescence studies, or arteriography may be helpful in evaluating erectile dysfunction but do not provide much diagnostic insight in the evaluation of PE itself. However, concerns about erectile dysfunction add to PE, so these tests may be important if you are experiencing both PE and erectile dysfunction.

If there are no identified physical causes, then review again the possibilities of other causes, especially psychological or relationship distress. Mixed PE commonly involves a deficit in psychosexual skills, and skills learning may become your treatment of choice. Cognitive behavioral sex therapy may also help remedy the detrimental effects of erectile dysfunction–induced PE on you and your relationship.

If you have PE with erectile dysfunction, oral medications and other erectile dysfunction treatments—vacuum constriction devices, intracavernous or intraurethral pharmacotherapy, and penile prostheses—can be valuable resources. If your PE is a symptom of and compensation for a fear of erectile dysfunction, treating the erectile dysfunction can, in turn, resolve your PE.

Treatments for Erectile Dysfunction

Since erectile dysfunction is the most common factor in mixed PE, let's take a look at the medical treatments currently available for this problem.

Oral Medications

Medications such as Viagra and Cialis help initiate and maintain erection by relaxing the corpus cavernosum smooth muscle in the penis. Such medications can be used for erectile dysfunction whether its cause is physical, psychological, or medication related, and they can relieve PE that results from overcompensation for fears of erectile dysfunction. Among the most common unwanted effects are headache, facial redness, indigestion, visual disturbances, and nasal congestion. Each of these effects occurs in approximately 10 to 15 percent of men.

Medications Applied to the Penis

Erectile dysfunction is sometimes treated with medication applied directly to the penis.

PGE1. The most commonly used is E1-prostaglandin (PGE1) or alprostadil, which the man injects into the base of the penis a few minutes before sexual activity. PGE1 may be used up to two to three times a week. When erection is assured by injection therapy, men with mixed PE may relax, thereby gaining control of ejaculation. However, many men stop using injection therapy because they or their partners find it awkward and clinical.

MUSE. Medicated Urethral System for Erection (MUSE) is a device used to insert an alprostadil suppository into the urethral opening. Reports of its effectiveness vary from 7 to 65 percent. The most common adverse effects are penile pain, urethral burning, dizziness, or fainting. MUSE may be more user-friendly than injection therapy, but it also has a very high dropout rate.

Vacuum Constriction Devices

Vacuum constriction devices draw blood into the penis, causing an erection, and trap the blood there in order to maintain the erection for intercourse. These devices include a plastic tube that fits over the penis in order to create an airtight cover. A vacuum is created around the penis by motor or manual pumping. When erection occurs by this means, a fitted rubber band is placed on the penis at the base to retain the erection. An erection may be maintained by this method for approximately thirty minutes. Again, there is a high dropout rate due to lack of comfort on the part of either the man or the woman.

Penile Prostheses

Nonsurgical prostheses include splints such as Rejoyn, a soft rubber brace which holds the flaccid penis rigid. The brace exposes the tip of the penis to allow for pleasure. Some women find the device uncomfortable during intercourse. These are available without prescription at many drugstores.

Rigid or flexible rods may be surgically implanted into the penis to make it mechanically erect. There are inflatable models that allow for artificial engorging and deflating of the penis by means of a hydraulic system composed of tubes implanted in the penis and a fluid reservoir or bulb implanted in one of the testicular sacks (the testis is removed). The tubes are then inflated by squeezing the bulb and deflated by a valve in the bulb. These surgeries do not allow for an actual erection, but do permit the penis to be comfortably inserted into the vagina. Because implants are irreversible and do not allow any other treatments, an implant is the last option for treating erectile dysfunction.

While these medical treatments are clearly helpful for many men with PE combined with erectile dysfunction, they each have significant limitations. These treatments succeed best when used along with the PE skills program and when integrated into a flexible style of couple sexuality that encompasses intimacy, pleasuring, and eroticism.

Your Body and Person Are Intertwined

When you suspect that medical problems are causing your PE, you need to carefully evaluate medical and physical resources. Approaching PE as a psychological or relationship problem without addressing the medical cause will lead to confusion, frustration, disappointment, and a sense of failure and hopelessness.

Your body and person are intrinsically intertwined. Appreciating and respecting that your personality is fundamentally grounded or housed in your body is important. With your body healed, or the reality of its limitations understood, you are ready to pursue the psychological and relationship skills to manage your PE and enhance your intimacy.

7

Psychological and Relational Strategies and Skills

David developed PE during the second year of his marriage to Kristin due to a mild prostate infection that was undetected and untreated for four years. Although they eventually learned that David's PE was caused by a medical problem, David and Kristin realized that the years of PE had cost them dearly. PE had played a substantial role in undermining David's self-esteem and confidence, causing sexual stress that injured their overall relationship.

During the four years that they endured the PE, David and Kristin became stressed and estranged by intense arguing and fighting—first about PE, and later about nonsexual issues. There were days when they avoided each other not only sexually but personally. The psychological distress he experienced with the recent death of his father also weighed on David. The combination of grieving and the relationship alienation caused by their arguing became a maintaining cause of PE, even after antibiotics had cured the prostate infection that initially caused the PE.

David and Kristin's distress wasn't limited to the bedroom—it permeated their entire relationship. To recover, they learned how to emotionally accept the hurt around their sexuality, how to heal the mutual pain, and how to resolve relationship conflict. David and

Kristin learned crucial skills for relationship intimacy: understanding and integrating relationship expectations, developing emotional empathy, and implementing mutual conflict resolution.

This chapter is designed to help you approach the psychological aspects of PE. This will be helpful to you if you have psychological system PE, psychological distress PE, relationship distress PE, or other types of PE that have caused distress to you and your relationship. You will learn an approach to address individual psychological features that cause, maintain, or result from PE. You'll also address distress in your relationship identity, relationship cooperation, or relationship intimacy that causes, maintains, or results from PE. We'll teach you skills to clarify your sexual relationship identity, modify your interaction dynamics, and emotionally support each other.

We'll describe specific ways to become more aware of your feelings and discuss the importance of investing emotionally in your relationship to promote healing and enhance empathy. We'll teach you a specific communication skill, *paraphrasing*, to make your emotional investment easier and safer, and we'll show you ways to cooperate and resolve disagreements. These skills will help you and your partner work as a team to learn ejaculatory control and enjoy sex.

Approaches to Relieve Individual Psychological Distress

In this section, we'll look at ways to approach PE caused by long-term or temporary individual psychological distress. With either type, you should remain open to evaluation and treatment for chemical dependency if you have been "medicating" yourself with alcohol or drugs. See the Resources section for more information.

Strategies to Resolve Psychological System PE

Psychological system PE is very difficult to address with self-help approaches. However, you can gain insight with basic information from a reliable book or a reputable Web site on the condition you suspect. Consultation with a licensed clinical psychologist can help you determine whether you have a chronic psychological problem that might cause your PE. Consultation usually includes one or more personal interviews, a historical review of your life, and some psychological testing.

Treatment for PE caused by a psychological problem may include individual or group psychotherapy, medication, and sex therapy. Because your psychological system is complex and tends to resist change, realize that it may take a considerable amount of time and effort in therapy to address the feature you believe is causing PE. When you feel ready, learn the psychosexual skills in chapter 8.

Shane's Story: Obsessive-Compulsive Disorder

Shane had frequently wondered how different his life might be without anxiety, hypersensitivity, perfectionism, and orderliness. He had never thought that his PE was related to these traits, because he had always ejaculated very fast. When life was particularly stressful, Shane noticed that he would act more ritualistically, compulsively checking whether the coffee pot was turned off or all doors were locked, ruminating about what seemed to be small concerns, and having trouble deciding to discard things. When it came to sex, he constantly felt stressed and anxious, believing he should "do sex perfectly."

When Shane consulted with a psychologist, he described the day-to-day features he suspected were obsessive-compulsive, reviewed his personal history, and completed a psychological test. The test results suggested that he did in fact have strong obsessive-compulsive personality features as well as anxiety traits, which supported the psychologist's diagnosis: obsessive-compulsive disorder (OCD).

Shane's treatment plan included learning about OCD by reading two books, extended individual therapy to explore the nature of his OCD and develop strategies to cope better, taking an SSRI medication (which not only alleviated his OCD but had the side-effect of slowing ejaculation), brief couple therapy to enlist his wife's acceptance and support, and finally couple sex therapy to learn psychosexual skills for slowing ejaculation. While Shane's treatment involved an extensive amount of time, he was able to make significant progress in altering his personal quality of life, overcoming PE, and enhancing relationship intimacy.

Strategies to Resolve Psychological Distress PE

If you indicated on your PE Diagnostic Summary Sheet in chapter 4 that you have psychological distress PE, review what you noted to be the stressors that cause your PE, as well as whether another type of PE might be causing psychological distress that worsens the sexual problem.

Most men prefer to address the specific psychological stressor using self-help efforts since this type of problem is less severe and chronic than psychological system PE. If self-help doesn't work for you, use good judgment and seek appropriate professional therapy.

As a couple, you want to discuss how best to address the sources of your psychological distress PE. For example, if you are stressed about career issues that—for the moment—you are not able to resolve, you may decide together to accept this temporary distress and compensate sexually by learning the skills in chapter 8. The important thing is that you pay attention to the underlying psychological distress causing your PE and make sure that you work together to prevent further problems.

Among your options, consider reading a reliable book or visiting a reputable Web site on the type of stress you suspect. There are a number of very good self-help books that can help you understand your distress, and offer practical suggestions for adapting (see Resources). If reading and reflecting on your circumstances is not your style, or if your self-help approach is not effective, you will benefit from talking with a psychologist. He or she can help you gain perspective on your distress, offer objective psychological testing, and help you consider further strategies for change. If marital issues are causing your psychological distress (for example, an affair has led to depression), this cause needs to be addressed. Medication may be beneficial in addressing depression or anxiety rooted in current stresses.

In some cases, resolution of the psychological problem will restore normal sexual function, while in others the exercises in chapter 8 or sex therapy may be needed to overcome secondary problems, factors such as anticipatory anxiety, performance anxiety, or loss of sexual confidence. These factors can maintain your PE even when the psychological cause has been resolved.

When Your Partner Is Psychologically Distressed

PE may be your reaction to your partner's psychological problem. In this case, your PE serves as a relationship symptom of her psychological distress. Her psychological distress can cause PE when you feel tension during lovemaking and your body reflexively responds with urgency to "get it over with." Depression, obsessive-compulsive disorder, mood disorders, career distress, role conflicts, sleep deprivation and fatigue, parenting stresses, family conflicts, grieving the loss of a parent, loneliness, acute anxiety, and other problems—even when mild—can subvert sexual enjoyment.

Treatment for her psychological distress is similar to what we outlined above. Your empathy and emotional support for her is important. Such distress is an opportunity to build deeper intimacy by cooperatively addressing the difficulty.

Approaches to Alleviate Relationship Distress

If you indicated on your PE Diagnostic Summary Sheet that you have relationship distress PE, take a moment to recall the interpersonal dynamics you believe might be causing or maintaining your PE. Even if you have another type of PE, your relationship may have suffered. You'll need to heal the hurt and restore relationship quality. This section will offer you an approach to address the most common cognitive, behavioral, and emotional features of relationship distress.

Your Partner's Dissatisfaction

Similar to the way your partner's psychological distress may be transmitted to your body and affect your ejaculatory control, you can emotionally sense your partner's relationship dissatisfaction. Even though you may feel satisfied with your relationship except for your PE, your partner may feel lonely or disconnected from you and long for more emotional intimacy. If your partner does feel dissatisfaction with your interactions, this may be a factor in causing your PE as well as a result of it. Ask her. You may want to avoid dealing with her disappointment, but it is important to know because it is important to address the problem.

Identifying Your Relationship Distresses

This exercise uses the identity-cooperation-intimacy model described in chapter 3 to help you identify your relationship distresses. Honestly answer the following questions, first individually, then as a couple.

EXERCISE: IDENTIFYING YOUR RELATIONSHIP DISTRESSES

1. Identity Concerns

Are you struggling over expectations or disagreements regarding gender roles, work and family commitments, day-to-day tasks, the role of sex in your relationship, parenting, or balancing your autonomy with cohesion as a couple? Do you feel an imbalance in your desire to please your partner to the point that you neglect your own wants?

2. Cooperation or Conflict Resolution Concerns

Do you feel your partner is demanding? Have you felt pressure to ejaculate quickly in order to "get it over with"? How competitive are you with each other? Are you ready to cooperate to do the skills training? Have you offered forgiveness of each other (and yourself) for the hurts? Can you be patient, warm, and kind with each other? Are the outcomes to your disagreements emotionally satisfying for each?

3. Emotional Intimacy Concerns

Have you been afraid of deeper intimacy or more solid closeness? Are there hidden hurts that linger due to unresolved relationship conflicts? Have you corrected any empathy deficits? Are you holding a grudge? Are you afraid you won't be able to change your relationship feelings? How lonely do you feel in your relationship?

Recovering and Promoting Relationship Satisfaction

To alleviate relationship distress PE, you will need to work on one or more of the following objectives:

- Identity: Clarify and integrate your relationship and sexual beliefs, standards, perceptions, attributions, and expectancies, and balance individual autonomy and couple bonding.

- Intimacy: Enhance your emotional empathy in order to heal relationship injuries caused by conflict or by your PE.

- Cooperation: Modify interpersonal dynamics that may cause or maintain your PE, such as communication deficits or a conflict resolution impasse.

Clarifying Your Relationship Identity

Your beliefs, standards, and expectations of yourself and your partner about how to be a couple make up your relationship identity, while your sexual relationship identity comprises your sexual beliefs, standards, and expectations. Differences and misunderstandings are to be expected; they are normal. Clarifying such misunderstandings and integrating your new understandings into your couple style is part of reducing relationship distress.

Consider your sexual relationship identity. What does sex mean to you? A source of emotional vitality? Procreation? Pleasure? Duty? Joy? What role should sex play in your relationship? Do you expect to talk openly of your sexual wants, dislikes, joys, comfort, ideas? Should your sex always be wild passion? Tender lovemaking? Do you agree that there is more than one kind of sex? (Quickies? Impulsive passion? Mechanical anxiety release? Romance?) Do you and your partner expect to take turns being "sexually selfish"? Do you expect sexual pleasure to decrease or increase over time? Are you sexually playful? Respectful? Tender? Can sex bring consolation during stressful periods? Although you have had problems, do you think sex can improve? Do you share a standard of good-enough sex?

Balancing Autonomy and Couple Cohesion

At their core, relationship identity issues are usually problems balancing individual autonomy and relationship cohesion. This can play out in the sexual relationship and in the relationship as a whole. The autonomy couple cohesion balance is the central feature of your relationship identity. It directly influences your feelings as a couple and forms the foundation for cooperation and intimacy—including sex.

EXERCISE: SEEKING BALANCE IN YOUR GENERAL RELATIONSHIP

Consider your thoughts and feelings about how well you are balancing your individuality and your relationship cohesion. Talk with your partner directly about what you believe a relationship should involve and how to "do" a satisfying relationship. What are your expectations about how to communicate, deal with conflicts, express affection? What do you each believe and feel about gender roles, the role of sex, family-of-origin learnings, parental modeling of marriage, prior relationship experiences, spiritual beliefs, career goals, friendships, loyalties, religion, leisure, and social activities? What do you bring to your relationship? What do you feel proud of? What does your partner bring to the relationship that you appreciate?

Discuss (seeking information, not argument) your thoughts and feelings about how well you each are doing with the amount of individuality in your relationship. Then discuss the level of union or togetherness. Do you feel as independent as you want? Free or constrained? Do you have your own activities, interests? How stifled do you feel? Do you have as much time for yourself as you think you need? Where is your place to be alone, "off duty"?

What expectations do you have for your relationship, and how well are these being met? How highly do you and your partner prioritize your relationship? How lonely do you feel? How important is your partner to you? You to your partner? Are you able to have sufficient time together? To what degree do you approach daily life with a couple or team mentality? Relationship identity is the environment in which your sexual relationship lives.

EXERCISE: SEEKING BALANCE IN YOUR SEXUAL RELATIONSHIP

Discuss your thoughts about balance in your sexual relationship. What does it mean to balance individuality and couple cohesion during sex? Is individuality selfish? Does cohesion seem confining, smothering, distracting? Does your sex always have to be raw and physically passionate or deeply personal and romantic? Sexually, what do you bring to your relationship? What are you proud of sexually? What does your partner bring to your sexual relationship that you appreciate? Share your thoughts. Your sexual relationship identity is founded upon who each of you is as a unique individual and what you bring to your sex life.

When you strike a mutually satisfying and sustainable balance between individuality and interpersonal cohesion, good-enough sex results. Each of you contributes to the well-being of your relationship, and your relationship contributes to your growth, development, and well-being as individuals.

Enhancing Emotional Intimacy

Emotions about your relationship are the "energy source" for your sexual feelings. When relationship distress infringes on this positive energy, sexual problems can result. Feeling resentful, rejected, or fearful of your partner undermines sexual energy. Sexual problems like PE can drain your emotional energy as a couple. To recover from distress associated with PE, you will want to take steps to enhance your feelings of being an intimate team. You will want to improve your ability to recognize and gently express your feelings, deepen your appreciation of your partner's feelings, and together experience emotional empathy. Accepting and embracing each other's emotions will provide the foundation for working as a team to learn the psychosexual skills in chapter 8.

Feelings Are Essential to Intimacy

We want to focus on your emotions in this chapter because feelings are not only signs of the distress caused by your PE but also a key to resolving your PE. Because your emotions are indispensable for achieving sexual satisfaction, it is crucial that you be aware of them and comfortable with them. Everyone who has a body has feelings, but we differ in our level of awareness and comfort. Some are very aware of their body's sensations and feelings and have elaborate words to express them. Others are aware of their feelings but have few words to describe them clearly, or have learned to not express them out of shame, fear, or sensitivity. Still others ignore their feelings, believing emotions interfere with adult living.

What Are Feelings?

Feelings can be confusing, distracting, irritating, or frustrating unless you understand what they are about. Because many people—especially men—rely on reason more than emotion for direction in life, feelings are often viewed as irritants, distractions, or even enemies. Basically, feelings are biochemical energies in your body in response to various situations, influenced by your past experiences and current thoughts. Feelings are not enemies at all; they offer you important information that your reason might overlook. Feelings offer data about yourself and your experiences that are not available to you from logic or thinking alone.

Feelings Can Be Complicated

Often we have "mixed feelings"—we feel two or more at the same time. For example, you may worry that PE is impossible to resolve, feel hurt and irritated at yourself or your partner, and feel shame that you have failed to find a resolution—all simultaneously.

You may focus on only one dimension of the energy (feeling) in your body, ignoring the other feelings. For example, focusing only on frustration, you may miss feelings of hurt and worry.

One feeling can be converted to another. A person who is taught to not feel anger may convert feelings of anger to shame. A person who is taught that anger is okay but fear isn't may feel angry when afraid or threatened.

Feelings Are Useful

People tend to think of feelings as positive or negative, good or bad, depending on whether they agitate (like fear, anger, and guilt) or encourage (like pleasure, contentment, and satisfaction). Our approach to understanding feelings is to think of them as voices trying to get your attention so you'll consider factors other than logic in your response to a situation. Feelings try to help you respond to different situations. Every feeling is good in terms of its purpose to serve you, protect you, and guide you. Your feelings offer honest information, some of which you may not like. Listening for feelings is an important skill.

Metaphors for Feelings

Consider two metaphors that a number of men and women have told us helped them appreciate the value of emotions.

Psychological sonar. As you navigate through life, you are continuously monitoring the environment for information about your situation. Imagine your logical reason to be your "psychological radar," supplying information about what is going on "aboveground." Then imagine that your emotional intelligence is your "psychological sonar," supplying information about what is going on "below the water." (If you are a sportsman, imagine the sonar fish finder in your boat.) Different systems offer different information, and the composite information from both radar and sonar offers you a more complete picture of your situation.

With PE, your "radar" or reason may have told you, "I will again fail to please her," while your "sonar" or emotions likely alerted you with anxiety and tension in your body. Both alert you in different ways to a challenging situation.

Lifelong, loyal friends. Another way to understand your feelings is to consider them to be your "buddies" or lifelong, loyal friends. They have been with you through your experiences, and they remember them even when you forget. Each feeling, then, is a savvy veteran of experience who will alert or protect you from situations that experience leads him to believe could distress you. Your friend vigilantly looks after you. He will not lie to you, abandon you, or be silent when concerned that you may forget or be misled by your logic. A good buddy will take you aside, counsel you, even argue with you when he thinks you could be making a mistake or overlooking potential trouble. You may not like the counsel of these friends, thinking they overprotect you or make things worse for you, but they are just doing their job whether you like it or not.

Suppose you have experienced your partner's disappointment when you ejaculated quickly and concluded that you were inadequate. You experienced intercourse as failure. Your loyal friends—your feelings of shame and anxiety—wanted to protect you from further failure, so they tried to get your attention and maybe even advised you to avoid sex.

EXERCISE: LISTENING FOR YOUR FEELINGS

Alone, provide yourself a quiet, relaxing atmosphere. Relax your body until you are feeling calm, centered, and comfortably aware of your body. Then imagine that you are a miniature explorer traveling around inside your body to find where different feelings are most strongly noticeable to you. Where in your body do you experience joyful feelings? In your face, eyes, mouth? In your chest or legs? Where in your body do you experience feelings of anxiety or fear? In your stomach? In your chest? In your cold hands? Where in your body do you experience anger? In your hot cheeks or ears? In your throat or neck? In your stomach? Where in your body do you experience feelings of sadness? Where in your body do you experience feelings of confusion, indecisiveness, ambivalence? Where in your body do you experience feelings of sensuality with your partner?

Write down what you learned.

Are You Free to Feel?

While your feelings are valuable sources of personal information, it's not always a good idea to act on them. Whether and how to act are ethical choices that you need to make. For example, a feeling of anger offers personal information to you about your situation, usually one in which you feel hurt, threatened, or blocked. Or, experiencing PE, you may feel frustrated. These feelings get your attention by agitating your body so you recognize the problem. What you do with this information is the ethical issue.

The guiding principle is this: Accept your feelings, judge your behaviors. When you make this distinction between your feelings and behaviors, you are free to feel. You can feel frustration about PE and choose not to express this feeling to your partner. Rather, you can choose a more positive course of action by asking your partner for a few moments to rest and recover, and then offering to pleasure her as she wishes. You want to learn from your feelings but not let them run your life; you don't have to act on them. You want to listen to your feelings, consider their counsel, and decide how to respond in a constructive fashion. Integrating your feelings and reason gives you a more complete picture of your situation.

Value Your Partner's Feelings

Accept your partner's feelings as well as your own. Accepting a feeling does not mean agreeing or condoning. It means listening, valuing, caring, accepting, affirming, and nurturing her. You can accept and affirm your partner's feeling of anger without agreeing with her interpretation (attribution) of the problem and without condoning the behaviors expressing anger. Don't try to "fix" or change your partner's feelings. Ironically, your acceptance is the major thing that will help your partner's feelings to change. Strive to acknowledge, affirm, and accept feelings.

Different Ways of Expressing Feelings

There are many direct and indirect ways to express feelings. The words to describe feelings are learned. Some words directly describe emotions: "I feel sad," "I feel warm and close," "I feel frustrated." Others express feelings indirectly. You might say, "Isn't it a nice day?" to express "I feel wonderful today" or say, "All you do is spend money" to mean "I am worried about money." The more directly you express your feelings, the more likely it is that your partner will understand and interpret your meaning correctly.

You and your partner have your own emotional language, nonverbal (a smile, a glance away) as well as verbal. How do you express your feelings? How does your partner? How have you expressed feelings about your PE? How has your partner? Verbally? Nonverbally? Negatively? Calmly? Dramatically? Developing healthier ways to share feelings is important and will deepen your intimacy. Learning to "read" your partner's words and actions is part of the uniqueness of intimacy. It takes months or years of sharing experiences, explaining to each other your thoughts and feelings, for better and for worse.

Communicating emotions is an important skill in an intimate relationship. For many men and women, it is difficult to feel close without sharing verbally what and how you feel. Love involves sharing warm, positive feelings and romance, but also involves sharing feelings even when that may lead to conflict. Communicating negative feelings in a positive, constructive way can lead to emotional closeness. You can still be loved and valued even if you are down, anxious, or had a failure experience. Love tries to provide that safe harbor amidst the storms of life.

Vulnerability within Emotional and Sexual Intimacy

Sharing your feelings with your partner is important to healing and deepening your long-term sexual relationship. Emotional openness and the nakedness of sex are the two most vulnerable and tender aspects of committed love. During these experiences, we are most exposed and fearful of rejection. You can appreciate your sensitivity when you consider how it hurt when you shared feelings and felt rejected or shamed. Or consider when you ejaculated quickly and felt sexually vulnerable but your partner seemed frustrated, misreading your distress as blame or abandonment. You probably wanted to hide your emotional vulnerability and cover up your physical nakedness. When you give and receive empathy while you are vulnerable emotionally and sexually, you communicate powerful acceptance and comfort, and generate trust and love.

EXERCISE: EXPRESSING FEELINGS AND EMOTIONS

If you have difficulty describing your feelings with words, use the same words over and over, or tend to confuse feelings with thoughts, you can fine-tune your skills with this couple exercise.

Below is a list of words that describe feelings or emotions. Add any favorites of your own or others you can think of. Then do the three "building blocks" that follow.

pleased	excited	comfortable
happy	jubilant	satisfied
glad	elated	contented
aroused	surprised	stimulated
confident	eager	peaceful
witty	joyful	calm
hopeful	playful	composed
fascinated	silly	thoughtful
angry	frightened	bored
provoked	anxious	weary
quarrelsome	afraid	apathetic
insulted	cowardly	complacent
irritated	cautious	tired
discontented	uneasy	worried
uncomfortable	hesitant	nervous
overwhelmed	ashamed	worthless
daring	energetic	embarrassed
intense	distracted	earnest
enraged	hurt	tender
confused	passionate	sad

Building block 1. Alone, take a moment to reflect and write down some notes on your experience. What words do you use most frequently to describe your feelings? What words do you hear your partner use most often? Do you and your partner have different favorite words to express a similar feeling? What are they? Which feelings are most familiar to you? What are your labels or words for these? What other feelings might be concealed behind these words? After you have finished your notes, spend at least ten minutes each sharing these with your partner.

Building block 2. For one full day, discuss with your partner your impressions as you observe each other giving nonverbal signals such as tone of voice, facial expressions, physical movements, and body positions. Tell each other what you interpret the other to be feeling. Share where you got your impression and check this out with each other. For example, "I see you chewing your nails and it makes me think you are feeling nervous. Am I right?" "I hear you talking very loudly and it makes me think you are feeling irritated. Are you?" "You are quiet. Are you feeling sad?" "I feel your arm around me and it makes me think you are feeling romantic. Do you want to make love?"

Building block 3. What words do you use most frequently to describe your sexual feelings? Like many men, you might use only one word, *good*. This doesn't give your partner much to go on, so think of additional descriptive words. What words do you hear your partner use most often? Do you and your partner have favorite words to express sexual feelings? What are they? Do you use words during sex that turn you on? Turn you off? Which words? What are your labels or names for each other's body parts? Do you have playful nicknames for these? What nonverbal signals do you use during lovemaking? How do you interpret your partner's tone of voice, facial expressions, and physical movements during sex? How does your partner interpret yours? Tell each other your impressions and check these out with each other.

The Emotional Skill, Empathy

In intimate relationships, an important ideal is to feel emotionally valued and accepted without conditions, to feel unconditional positive regard from and for each other. Empathy, the skill of affirming feelings, is the glue of your relationship. It feels good to have your successes and strengths accepted, but you feel especially loved and respected when your vulnerabilities and weaknesses are embraced. To empathize with your partner, imagine for a moment that you are her. You imagine that you think and feel as she does, that you experience her reality. When you are empathic with your lover, you offer the greatest gifts: acceptance, nurturance, warmth, respect, reassurance, validation, care, patience, and appreciation. These are wonderful qualities to take into the bedroom!

Modifying Your Relationship Dynamics

Changing the relationship dynamics involved in your PE will require effective communication and mutual conflict resolution. We'll begin by teaching paraphrasing, a communication skill which helps develop the emotional skill of empathy.

Paraphrasing

Paraphrasing helps you clarify your relationship identity and bring your intentions and your partner's perceptions in line. This cognitive congruence is the foundation for emotional empathy. With careful use of paraphrasing, you and your partner will achieve clarity of communication, emotional empathy, and readiness for mutual conflict resolution. Here's how it works:

1. "I" message. Partner 1 reveals himself by expressing his thoughts and feelings, trying to be clear, direct, and open as he shares his personal message. The focus is on him only. He says, "I think . . . ," "I feel. . . ." This is a personal disclosure or sharing, an opening of his heart. Partner 2 may nod or say "uh-huh" but not interrupt.

2. Paraphrase. Partner 2 listens with undivided attention, then summarizes the "I" message in her own words, stating her understanding of what Partner 1 has shared. The paraphrase begins, "What I think I hear you saying is. . . ." Her focus is solely upon him. Paraphrasing is empathetic listening—offering in her own words her understanding of his thoughts and feelings.

3. Appraisal. Partner 1 then evaluates their effort for empathetic understanding. He asks himself, "As I listen to her paraphrase, am I feeling completely understood?" If he feels a full empathetic understanding, then the appraisal is yes. If not, the appraisal is no.

4. If the appraisal is no, Partner 1 begins the cycle again, fine-tuning his "I" message.

There are two ways to use paraphrasing: two-way or "leapfrog" paraphrasing, where partners switch roles when a yes appraisal verifies empathy, and one-way or single-focus paraphrasing, where the partners do not switch roles after a yes appraisal, allowing the same partner to continue. One-way paraphrasing offers the partner with several urgent messages the opportunity to continue working until satisfied.

The appraisal step empowers you by assuring that you will be understood to your satisfaction, or discussion does not go further. When it is your "I" message, you have the control to guarantee you receive empathy. A yes appraisal means "I certify that you understand me now because I have heard and felt your empathy." When the feeling being shared is complicated, it is reasonable to need ten, twenty, or more "I" messages before the empathy is confirmed with a yes. The first few "I" messages typically focus on describing the content, and subsequent "I" messages focus on clarifying the quality of your feelings about the content.

Paraphrasing will provide you the discipline and patience to yield profound understanding. Your patience with the process demonstrates that you value your partner's feelings. Paraphrasing is particularly valuable for talking about your sexual feelings. It provides you a system to talk with understanding and appreciation.

EXERCISE: PARAPHRASING

Take fifteen minutes to practice communicating using the two-way paraphrasing format. At first, be very disciplined, saying nothing outside the structure. Let the man begin with an "I" message. It will help if you make an audiotape of your practice. Afterward, review your audiotape together. If you have practiced with discipline, notice that you can talk together calmly because the format gives you control over the communication process. Notice that if you are loyal to the paraphrasing discipline, you cannot have an argument! The structure prevents it. You now have a format to achieve emotional empathy.

Using Your New Skills to Recover Emotionally from PE

Your new skills at empathizing and paraphrasing provide a powerful foundation for overcoming the emotional hurt of PE. You can now look at PE as an opportunity to grow together as a couple. When you feel accepted and respected even if you "fail" sexually, you develop a special bond with your partner. When you understand that your partner felt hurt and abandoned because she assumed that you valued sexual performance over personal intimacy, your bond is deepened. Take the opportunity. Paraphrase your feelings.

There is no real love without hurt, pain, suffering, and disappointment. Normal day-to-day limitations to affection, occasional misunderstandings and hurts, occasional mediocre sex, personal imperfections: these are common relationship disappointments. Acceptance—or at least tolerance—of such vicissitudes of life is important for forgiveness. Regardless of its cause, your PE warrants compassion and kindness from and for each other.

Forgiveness requires you to expand your understanding of what PE means for each of you and to strengthen your relationship cohesion with empathetic communication. By discovering each other's intentions and perceptions, you can change your perspective, not looking backward but looking to the future. Learning to redefine the sexual component of your intimate relationship while you learn the practical lovemaking skills to overcome PE will solidify your forgiveness and healing as lovers.

Renewal of intimacy requires honest acceptance that there has been hurt in the past. These feelings do not need justification; they are simply your loyal friends letting you know that aspects of sex have been unsatisfying. It is essential to heal the emotional pain because your relationship feelings are the energy source for your sexual relationship.

Cooperation for Conflict Resolution

Most relationship disagreements or "fights" ultimately stem from hurt feelings or a failure to share emotional empathy. Conflict remains unresolved when partners reach an impasse in their efforts to communicate effectively and empathetically to resolve differences. If fighting has caused your PE, or if PE has caused fights, notice that your lack of empathy for each other's hurt and confusion was an important issue, maybe even more important than sexual function. Even relatively minor behavioral conflicts like tidiness and punctuality can flare and become major emotional arguments when each partner feels rejected. The skill of cooperation is required to resolve conflicts in mutually satisfying ways.

Understanding Relationship Conflict and PE

The role of relationship conflict in PE is important because the way you resolve differences—including sexual differences—either builds or diminishes intimacy.

To discover the role of relationship conflict in your experience of PE, try the following exercise. Go on a fact-finding mission.

EXERCISE: WHERE, WHEN, HOW, AND WHY DO YOU FIGHT?

1. Where and when do you fight? When you have nonsexual conflicts, consider where you typically are and when the conflict

occurs. What are the patterns of your conflict? Do you tend to fight on particular days? At particular times of the day? What happens before the conflict—what circumstances seem to set the stage? For example, you might argue while driving home after visiting your mother, or in the bedroom Saturday night after your teenager misbehaves and after you have been drinking. Who else is present or nearby when you have conflict? How long does the disagreement typically last? What happens after the disagreement? There may be individual issues that you bring to your relationship that create the environment for the conflict. What unsettling events in the past might have influenced the way you and your partner approach conflict resolution in the present? When you understand that conflict may be linked to particular situations, you can anticipate and regulate conflict more effectively.

In your sexual relationship, consider these same questions. What are the patterns of conflict in response to PE?

2. What do you do when you fight? Consider how you respond to each other when disagreement occurs. Do you cooperate, confront, act playfully? Yield, evade, withdraw? If another person was watching, what would that person see you doing? How do you perceive that your partner feels and behaves when you disagree?

When PE occurs, how does each of you respond? With shame? Caring? Irritability? Tears? Withdrawal? Criticism? Are these responses helpful? Constructive?

3. What does conflict mean? Why are you fighting, and what does the disagreement mean to you? What thoughts typically go through your mind about your partner and about the conflict? What part of the conflict do you react most strongly to? What do you think causes the conflict? What is upsetting to you about the fact that you and your partner have a conflict in this particular area? Do your conflicts reflect different beliefs about how your relationship should be? What do you expect will result when the two of you discuss important relationship topics? What would you like to see happen? What would calm you or make you feel satisfied?

Now, review these same questions as you focus specifically on PE. Why is PE so painful? What are your thoughts and feelings? What does PE represent or mean to each of you?

What you learn from these reflections will help you to better understand your beliefs about conflict, your perceptions and attributions, and the meaning of your conflict. This knowledge can help you work out mutual solutions to your disagreements and motivate you to work as a team to resolve your PE.

Conflict Is an Opportunity for Intimacy

While many couples view disagreements as threats to their intimacy, in truth, addressing conflict or discord is the ordinary process through which couples deepen their intimacy. When each partner engages in a dispute with the goal of prevailing in what he or she wants, the other partner feels unimportant, disregarded, and rejected. However, with cooperation and mutual empathy, partners learn to understand the meaning and deeper feelings behind the conflict. Then both can participate in finding a mutually satisfying resolution. The guiding principle is that each partner must feel emotionally satisfied with the outcome.

Win-win solutions are not always achievable. When this is the reality, couples are confronted with the need to accept their differences. Most couples are capable of achieving this when they feel a sense of equity about who is doing the compromising. Integration of differences is ideal; acceptance is satisfying; toleration is adequate.

Resolving Conflict Mutually

To mutually resolve conflicts—including conflicts about PE—you need to cooperate to do the following:

- Be willing to vulnerably invest your thoughts and feelings in your relationship.

- Apply self-discipline and leadership, and use structured communication—paraphrasing—to ensure that your intentions and your partner's perceptions are congruent.

- Use paraphrasing to generate emotional empathy.

- Formulate the issue or conflict as a couple problem. Address PE as "our" problem. Ask yourselves, "How do we resolve this problem in such a way that we both feel good about it?"

- Create a *mosaic* solution. The great majority of mutual solutions are mosaic solutions, meaning that they are made up of several specific behaviors which each partner contributes to the resolution. Such solutions feel good for both partners. Avoid either-or solutions, since they create a winner and loser. The steps in chapter 8 will offer ways to develop your mosaic sexual solution for PE.

- After you implement your resolution, evaluate it several days or weeks later to discuss how well it is working. Consider ways to strengthen it.

A system of mutual conflict resolution clarifies and integrates relationship identity through effective communication, which promotes satisfying conflict resolution (cooperation), which facilitates empathy (intimacy), which in turn supports relationship identity, and this positive cycle continues. This cognitive, emotional, and behavioral integration forms the healthy relationship foundation for you to overcome PE.

8

Psychosexual Skills: Enjoying Arousal and Regulating Orgasm

Mark and Lisa had been trying to remedy PE for more than six years. They had read everything they could find about PE and had tried every do-it-yourself technique, but nothing had really worked. Mark's family physician had agreed to prescribe a lidocaine anesthetic, which helped some, but Mark found it dissatisfying because he lost much of the feeling in his penis and felt even further alienated from his body. Lisa had tried to be passive during lovemaking, saying little and avoiding touching Mark so as not to overexcite him. She even expressed her dissatisfaction, trying to tone down his excitement. Lisa appreciated Mark's efforts, but still privately resented the PE.

Over the years, Mark and Lisa had found the problem more and more divisive, and they rarely talked of their feelings about PE—only about what to do to fix it. Mark became more and more preoccupied with his "failure" to perform, and over time he began to avoid sex, anticipating that he would come fast and worrying that he could not please Lisa. Lisa began to feel Mark was more concerned about his penis and performance than about her. There were periods when Mark would come fast, feel frustrated and irritated, apologize to Lisa or berate himself for being "messed up," and then leave the bedroom. Lisa felt more and more abandoned by Mark as their sexual interaction progressively worsened. It was hard for her to not react angrily herself. It was all such a disappointment.

Lisa and Mark felt hopeless. Their efforts had brought no significant changes. They were, in fact, doing worse and feeling more and more alienated from each other. They felt inadequate, isolated, and inferior to other couples who didn't have sex problems. They had read that PE was the easiest male sex problem to correct, which deepened their frustration and shame. Lisa felt angry that Mark would not seek help from a professional sex therapist. Mark felt that sex was too private, and he doubted that therapy could help. Chronic PE was harming their overall marital relationship, limiting their communication, and testing their emotional support of each other. They were in marital as well as sexual trouble.

Mark and Lisa did eventually go to sex therapy, but only after Lisa became so frustrated that she threatened to divorce Mark if he didn't "get his problem fixed." Lisa was hurt that it took such a severe threat to get Mark to act. It was hard for her to recognize his avoidance as a measure of how deep his shame was.

With the help of their sex therapist, Dr. Hernandez, Mark and Lisa began to comprehensively address the problem. Because their case was severe (they had a PESI score of 75), they needed to complete a very detailed series of steps to remedy both the PE and the damage to their relationship. Dr. Hernandez used a diagnostic process like the one outlined in chapter 4 to help Mark determine that his PE was caused by neurologic system predisposition and psychosexual skills deficit, and that the harm PE had already caused to the intimate relationship was also serving to maintain PE. Mark decided he did not want to take medication, so Dr. Hernandez helped them outline a strategy to compensate for the neurologic quickness and the skills deficit by cooperatively improving their psychosexual skills. The early sessions of therapy worked to heal the marital harm that had occurred.

In this chapter, we'll teach you the psychosexual skills to address PE. You'll learn to relax and regulate your arousal. You and your partner will learn to cooperate in ways that will provide sexual and relationship support, safety, and comfort. We'll provide detailed instructions every step of the way. We'll show you how Mark and Lisa gradually overcame PE, and how you can overcome it too. You will be amazed that PE can be effectively managed. You will not only last longer but enjoy significantly more pleasure, emotional connection, and intimacy.

How to Approach Learning the Psychosexual Skills

We'll begin by giving you an overview of the skills so you understand clearly what you are trying to achieve with each skill, how each skill relates to the others, and how to put the skills together.

Understanding the Four Phases of Skills Learning

There are eleven steps to learning the psychosexual skills, and these steps can be divided into four phases. As you work through the steps, be sure you understand the goal for each phase so that the exercises make sense.

Phase One: Comfort and Relaxation

The first series of exercises promotes comfort with your sexuality as an individual and couple, and teaches you individual cognitive and behavioral skills for relaxing your body. The essential skill is to focus on physical sensations in order to relax your body. This will help you pace your arousal.

Phase Two: Pleasure Toleration

In phase two, you'll work together as an intimate team to stay relaxed with increasingly more erotic stimulation. By focusing on relaxation, you will learn that you can welcome more—not less— pleasure without ejaculating. The essential skill is to tolerate increasingly intense pleasure without stepping off into ejaculatory inevitability.

Phase Three: Pleasure Saturation

In phase three, you'll learn how to have extended intercourse. The exercises will teach you how to begin intercourse, and then how to extend the closeness. You'll learn to enjoy intercourse, saturating yourselves with pleasure. The essential skill is integrating the cognitive and behavioral skills to manage PE during intercourse.

Phase Four: Long-Term Satisfaction

In the final phase, you will meld the psychosexual skills with the psychological and relationship aspects into your couple sexual style. The essential skill is integrating the multidimensional features to overcome PE as an intimate team, and to ensure long-term satisfaction with a sensible relapse prevention plan.

This chapter will guide you through the first three phases. Chapters 9 and 10 will guide you through phase four.

How to Tailor Your Steps to Your Level of Severity

Work with your partner to decide what steps fit your situation best. If you are recovering from PE caused by a medical, psychological, or relationship problem (and these have been treated), or your PE severity is mild, discuss together whether you want to do all the steps or only those that you think will help you recover. For example, if your PE was caused by a prostate infection, you likely do not need to learn every skill; instead, the pelvic muscle (PM) control training (step three), relaxed couple pleasuring (step six), and the intimate intercourse technique (step ten) may be enough to help you recover. If you have moderate PE (PESI 50–70), completing most of the eleven steps will probably resolve your PE if you choose your course judiciously. For example, in phase two, pleasure toleration, you may elect to bypass step eight, the individual stop-start pacing exercise, and concentrate instead on learning step nine, the couple stop-start pacing exercise. If your PESI severity score was severe (greater than 70), you will need to complete every exercise. The most reliable approach is to complete all of the steps; however, if you elect to not learn some steps and your program does not bring about the results you want, you can retrace your steps and complete them all, or you can consult a sex therapist for help. The more severe your PE, the more likely working with a marital and sex therapist will be helpful.

What If You Experience Distress during an Exercise?

Because you're trying to extend your skills and comfort level, some of these exercises may bring mild discomfort or anxiety. This is to be expected. However, should any of these exercises cause significant distress or discouragement (which is the opposite of what we want for you), be wise: protect yourselves from unintended hurt by seeking professional coaching and support.

The Psychosexual Skills: The Nitty-Gritties for Success

As they worked through the psychosexual skills, Mark and Lisa learned a reasonable way of thinking about PE and a realistic approach to changing it. They learned the importance of physiological relaxation, the importance of accepting personal responsibility, and the skill of cooperating by giving and receiving pleasure.

Mark and Lisa were challenged by the amount of discipline required, but they gradually gained confidence and began to see success. Lisa especially enjoyed sensual experiences which not only slowed the touching process but felt like a more genuine, meaningful connection with Mark. Working together helped them to feel closer as a couple.

During the process, if either became confused, they reminded each other of the larger goal: relationship closeness, with cooperation as the best way to accomplish this. Mark found it helpful to remember that physical relaxation was the essential strategy, and discovered that he could achieve this by focusing on the sensations in his body.

Dr. Hernandez encouraged Mark and Lisa to acknowledge the difficult aspects of learning the psychosexual skills. At first, the exercises seemed a huge intrusion into lovemaking—too mechanical and impersonal. Mark and Lisa accepted this, reminding themselves that they would eventually develop a more personalized couple sexual style.

Dr. Hernandez also coached Mark and Lisa to handle unintended ejaculation during any of the steps by staying focused on the effort. He suggested that Mark simply acknowledge the mistake by saying "oops" or "a work in progress," then pause thirty to sixty seconds before continuing. Mark was not to get sidetracked by sulking or apologizing. Mark discovered that when he did ejaculate unintentionally, it was because he lost focus on his physical sensations, was not sufficiently relaxed, or had miscalculated how well he was doing the particular step.

Finally, Dr. Hernandez told Mark and Lisa that if either thought things weren't going well during an exercise, they should simply ignore this, focus on the physical sensations involved, and wait until after they completed the exercise to discuss their perceptions. Dr. Hernandez suggested that Mark and Lisa thank each other after each session, no matter how poorly it might have seemed to go. The guideline: Deeply appreciate your partner's support and effort, and say so.

Phase One: Comfort and Relaxation

The exercises in phase one help increase your sexual self-esteem, teach you several fundamental arousal management skills, and enhance your sexual comfort as a couple by inviting you to share your sexual feelings. Learning body relaxation will provide the foundation for later steps, and will help counter the performance anxiety that accompanies PE. You will learn to become sensuously and sexually aroused while maintaining physiological relaxation.

Step One: Affirming Your Sexuality and Increasing Couple Sexual Comfort

Goal: Develop acceptance of your body and of sex, and develop openness with your partner

Mark and Lisa found that affirming their sexuality and enjoying sexual comfort helped them heal emotionally and broke the barriers of cautiousness and apprehension that had developed between them because of PE. Through this step, each worked to feel positive about his or her body and about sex, and they were able to discuss their motivations and feelings about their sexual experiences.

Positive Body Image

Scientific research consistently finds that sexual satisfaction is strongly related to how proud, self-respectful, and comfortable you are with your body, nudity, and touch. This is why a healthy, positive attitude toward sexuality is so important. If you don't have positive feelings about your body, other good things are stifled, especially your ability to physiologically relax and focus on sensuality.

Body self-acceptance may be difficult in our glamour-conscious culture, but it is an important component in self-esteem and is essential to intimate lovemaking. Worrying about your body's attractiveness is a major distraction. Remember that distraction contributes to sexual dysfunction. Your negative thoughts about your body ("I'm fat," "My stomach is too puffy," "I don't like the way my penis looks") are distractions.

We all have expectations about our sexual selves that are unrealistic and self-defeating. It is important to honestly examine your feelings about your body. There are some things you can change for the better and other things you must simply accept and live with.

INDIVIDUAL EXERCISE: BODY IMAGE AWARENESS

Set aside private, quiet, comfortable time for yourself. It is best to use a full-length mirror for this exercise. First, bring yourself to a state of calm and centeredness. Focus on your body. Begin by undressing in front of the mirror, and be aware of the way your body looks in various stages of dress and undress. When you are completely nude, stand in front of the mirror and examine your body in minute detail. Really look. Make eye contact. Be with yourself in the mirror. Survey your entire body.

Talk to yourself as you progress. Say out loud how you honestly feel about various aspects of your body. Include each little scar, mole, wrinkle, and pimple. You can exaggerate your feelings. Be loud about those parts that disgust you and exclaim proudly your feelings about the parts you like. Move around, and watch your body as you change postures. Notice your muscles tense up, and notice your soft parts. Flex your muscles, pose, turn, dance, move seductively. Be aware of those parts of yourself that you usually avoid looking at: bulging stomach, small chest, skinny legs. Try to see these parts of yourself with some acceptance and a positive attitude. Integrate them into your view of your entire body.

Below are questions you might consider while you are doing this exercise.

- What do you like best about your body? What are you most proud of? How do you show this to your partner?

- How do you feel when your partner touches or looks at the parts of your body that you feel good about, proud of, and pleased with?

- What do you like least about your body? What are you ashamed of? How do you hide these parts of yourself? Do you avoid looking at them? Do you focus a lot of attention and self-criticism on them?

- How do you feel when your partner looks at or touches the parts of your body you don't like or feel ashamed of?

- How can you affirm your body and your physical self-image each day? Each time you make love?

Take a moment to consider what you can do to help yourself feel more confidence in your body. You might get a haircut, buy a piece of clothing that makes you feel sexy, or commit to getting in shape. Let it be something that helps you feel like your new, sexier self.

Couple Sexual Comfort

Sexual comfort feels good and creates an atmosphere in which you can learn the skills successfully. Partners who accept each other's shyness and even embarrassment with nudity, and who learn more about each other's personal thoughts and feelings toward their bodies and sexuality, feel more comfortable together. It was essential for Mark and Lisa to know that they could express their sexual feelings and be met with acceptance, respect, and caring.

You and your partner can develop increased sexual comfort by talking gently and openly about your positive sexual thoughts, feelings, wishes, and desires, as well as your sexual discomforts and inhibitions. Your sexual feelings are deeply personal and significant, so they deserve respect and tender care.

COUPLE EXERCISE: TALKING WITH YOUR PARTNER ABOUT SEXUAL FEELINGS

With mutual acceptance, take time to share your thoughts about the following.

Talk first about what you learned about sexuality as a child and adolescent. What did you learn about masturbation, marriage, petting, intercourse, oral sex, orgasm, how a man or woman was supposed to act during sex? Who taught you this? Talk about what it meant to you at the time as well as now.

What are your attitudes or beliefs about sexuality? What is okay and what is not okay during lovemaking? What do you *believe* is okay but don't *feel* is okay? What do you believe about intercourse? Oral sex? Anal intercourse? Experimentation? Sharing sexual fantasies? What do you believe about masturbation? Masturbating privately? With your partner's awareness? Without your partner knowing? Stimulating yourself while your partner watches? Mutual manual stimulation (simultaneously or taking turns)?

Talk about what you sexually like and appreciate about your partner.

Talk about how you feel about what you do together sexually. What do you really like about sex with each other?

Discuss with your partner sexual concerns you have, remembering to speak empathetically, warmly, and respectfully.

Share what you are feeling as you discuss your sexual thoughts, feelings, and beliefs. How does it feel to talk about sex?

Mark and Lisa found the body awareness exercise and talking about sex particularly helpful. Mark realized that his shyness about his body contributed to his anxiety during sex and made it difficult to relax. He also became more aware of his pleasure in touching Lisa, which allowed him to feel close to her. Lisa learned she felt conflicted about her body—she liked her face, eyes, and breasts, but felt her legs were ugly. She also shared that as a young girl she had been taught that sex was bad and still felt that intercourse was dirty. She even wondered if her discomfort somehow encouraged Mark to ejaculate quickly to get it over with. Such open discussions facilitated their comfort. Paradoxically, Mark worried that because this openness made him feel more sexually attracted to Lisa, it would make the PE worse. Dr. Hernandez reassured Mark that feeling attraction and comfort was healthy, and that he would learn how to enjoy this feeling in subsequent steps.

Step Two: Training Your Mind and Body for Relaxation

Goal: Learn relaxation, the foundation for ejaculatory control and pleasure

Satisfying sexual functioning depends on physical relaxation. You can't duck or bypass this skill if you're going to control ejaculation! We'll teach you to relax in your body, as opposed to the more common out-of-body relaxation strategies which focus on calm images (natural beauty) or soothing sounds (ocean waves). In-body relaxation helps eliminate performance anxiety and helps you focus on the physical sensations of pleasure. This body-focused relaxation is the foundation for sensual self-entrancement arousal. This is where your mental focus needs to be.

How to Handle Distractions

As you do the activities in this step, notice that when you try to focus on physical sensations, your mind may wander or jump to other places (work, kids, shopping, sports) 50 percent or more of the time. That's okay at first. Remember, this is a skill! If you didn't need to develop it, it would be automatic.

When you notice you are distracted, don't fight with the distraction or try to bulldoze it out of your mind. That just makes it worse. Take a moment to simply accept the distraction. Say hello to it; acknowledge it. This is important because every distraction has an emotional piece to it, a tiny energy of pressure or urgency. There is an emotional nudge to attend to it. If you ignore or fail to acknowledge the distraction, it will get stronger and will become a bigger distraction, pestering you for attention (remember that the function of a feeling is to get your attention). Talk to it for a moment so it knows you're paying attention, then gently set it aside until later.

You might imagine you see the distraction on your computer screen and then calmly press the "sleep" key to clear the screen. Or imagine you place the distraction in a file folder labeled "do later." Then calmly bring your attention back to the bodily sensation you are focusing on. At first, you will be spending a lot of time calming distractions, but gradually you'll find it easier to focus on the physical sensations. When you're focused on sensations more than 80 percent of the time, that's good enough!

INDIVIDUAL EXERCISE: PHYSICAL RELAXATION

Make yourself very comfortable in a chair, sofa, or bed, loosening any tight clothing. Close your eyes and relax. Breathe deeply and slowly: gradually inhale as you slowly count to five, then exhale to the count of five. Concentrate on feeling the air move slowly in and out of your body.

Concentrate on your toes. Relax them. Feel all the tension leave your toes. Breathe calmly, deeply. Relax your feet. Let all the tension in your feet disappear. Now let the tension in your calves disappear. Breathe slowly, deeply. Imagine a soothing feeling rising through your legs, through your knees to your thighs. Let your legs feel completely relaxed and free of tension. Breathe calmly, deeply, and feel the air glide through you.

Now focus on your pelvis. Let the muscles relax and let go of tension. Let this soothing feeling move through your buttocks; feel your buttocks relax. Feel yourself breathing deeply as the tension in the lower half of your body disappears. Then let the tension in your back begin to disappear. Let this soothing feeling wrap around your chest, shoulders, neck, down your arms and hands. Let this soothing feeling move through your face. Feel your facial muscles relax as you breathe calmly. Feel the tension disappear from your forehead, eyebrows, jaws. Just rest and allow your body and mind to feel relaxed and comfortable.

Although this is essentially an individual exercise, you and your partner can do it side-by-side. Lisa and Mark found it helpful to make an audiotape (about five minutes long) of these directions. By listening to the tape, they could concentrate more easily. They did the relaxation exercise seven times. This was good enough, and they were ready to move to step three.

Step Three: Learning Pelvic Muscle Control

Goal: Identify and learn to consciously control your pelvic muscle

This is the "don't be a tight ass if you want to control ejaculation" skill. It is common for your body to tighten in response to the pressures, tensions, and burdens of life. This includes unconsciously tightening your pelvic muscle (PM). By learning to relax it, you give yourself a premier technique to slow down ejaculation.

Pelvic Muscle Training

The easiest way to locate the PM is to imagine you are squeezing off urination or "twitching" your penis. You'll feel a mild sensation in one or more of the following areas: your penis, groin, the perineal area (between your testicles and anus), the gluteus maximus (butt) muscles, or the anus. Because the PM is muscle tissue, it can be conditioned or trained to perform more efficiently. What follows is a typical experience for many men, but your body may vary, so experiment to find what works for you.

The PM is used in two ways. First, because total body relaxation is the foundation for good ejaculatory control, attention to relaxing the PM during sexual activity is an efficient way to relax your whole body. If your PM relaxes, your whole body will follow. Second, when you keep your PM relaxed, the muscles involved in ejaculation are relaxed, reserved, or held back. Otherwise, you'd be "priming the pump" of ejaculation by reflexively tightening the PM during sexual excitement.

INDIVIDUAL EXERCISE: PM BASIC TRAINING

This exercise will improve your conscious awareness of the sensations of your PM and strengthen the muscle. Contract or tighten your PM and hold for three seconds, then relax it for three seconds while you continue to consciously focus on the sensations. Do this ten times—tightening three seconds, relaxing three seconds—for a total of one minute.

Do this set (contracting and relaxing the PM ten times) at three different times every day. At first it may be difficult to tighten and hold the muscle for three full seconds, but do what you can (one or two seconds) and build up your strength over time. When this is easy, move on to the next exercise.

INDIVIDUAL EXERCISE:
THE PM CONTINUUM

This exercise will increase your awareness of the sensation of your PM and increase your mental control of your PM. Visualize that your PM can be tightened in varying degrees of intensity, not simply tight or relaxed. Imagine a continuum from 1 to 10, at first with three marks: 1 (relaxed), 5 (medium), and 10 (tight). Practice moving from one point to another, holding the PM at that level for three seconds, then relax. For example, tighten the PM to 10 and hold for three seconds, then return to 1 for three seconds, then tighten to 5 and hold for three seconds, and then relax to 1. Practice this until it becomes easy. Once you learn this, extend the continuum from three stopping points to five stopping points (10—1—5—1—7—1—3—1). This will be good enough.

Step Four: Cognitive Pacing with the Sexual Arousal Continuum

Goal: Broaden the range of your sexual arousal

The PM training is a behavioral pacing skill. Next we'll show you how to develop a sexual arousal continuum as a foundation for your cognitive pacing skills. This continuum will be crucial when you learn progressive intercourse in step eleven.

Each of us has our own sexual arousal patterns or desired sequences that blend reality and imagination and facilitate sexual arousal. By understanding the level of arousal evoked by specific images, behaviors, and feelings, you can consciously modify eroticism in order to slow down, hold steady, or intensify arousal. In order to do so, you must develop awareness of how calming or stimulating a specific image, feeling, or behavior is for you.

INDIVIDUAL EXERCISE: DEVELOPING
YOUR OWN AROUSAL CONTINUUM

Make a detailed, specific list of images, feelings, behaviors, techniques, and scenarios that you find arousing. Using a scale of 1 to 100, with 100 equaling ejaculation or orgasm, assign an arousal level to each. In his list, Mark rated closed-lip kissing 20, fondling Lisa's breasts with clothes on 35, Lisa gently stroking his penis 60, fondling her naked breasts while Lisa gently stroked his penis 75.

Developing his detailed continuum taught Mark awareness of the arousal value of various sensual and sexual activities. It took him a number of weeks to fully delineate this continuum (he eventually distinguished more than forty specific focal points). This cognitive awareness created a powerful pacing technique that he later used to regulate his arousal during intercourse with Lisa.

Mark found that the things that occurred to him first were all highly arousing behaviors and images: focus on Lisa's breasts and genitals, oral sex, and intercourse—all items above 50. It was challenging for him to develop the 1 to 50 range of arousal items. Lisa also developed her continuum, and Mark learned that she found the opposite was true for her arousal pattern. She focused first on nongenital scenarios and found it more challenging to list the more arousing items. As they each completed an arousal continuum, Mark and Lisa talked openly of what they most enjoyed, which enhanced their sexual anticipation.

Step Five: Maintaining Relaxation during Arousal

Goal: Learn to combine relaxation and sensual self-entrancement arousal

This exercise will show you how easy it is to get an erection, let it subside, and regain it when you stay relaxed and focus on self-entrancement arousal. It is particularly helpful for men who also worry about erection problems. You'll want to practice this exercise several times. The first times you do this exercise, your goal is to relax and touch yourself without getting an erection. Then patiently allow an erection with the minimum of touch. Then you'll practice getting, losing, and regaining a relaxed erection.

INDIVIDUAL EXERCISE: RELAXED SELF-ENTRANCEMENT AROUSAL

In a private place, remove all your clothes and gently massage your body all over for fifteen minutes. Do not pursue arousal. Use this time to focus on your body's sensations to help you relax.

As you touch your entire body, be aware of the feeling of your skin and your hands on your skin. Try different kinds of touch: softer and harder, tickling or scratching, pinching lightly, fingering. Notice which feels better and where. Be aware of your body's contours: the soft, fatty parts; the bony parts; the firm, muscled parts. Be aware of the different textures of your skin—coarse, soft, smooth, hairy—and how each feels different to your hand. Try to notice your emotional reactions as well. Then, for another fifteen minutes, progressively do each of the following parts.

1. Soothing Genital Touch

After soothing your whole body for fifteen minutes, begin exploring your testicles and penis with very soft and slow touch. Do not use the intense stroking that you would with masturbation. Instead, concentrate on the quiet, calm sensations. Relax your PM and keep it relaxed. For at least five minutes, use featherlike touching or fingering to explore your sensations without getting an erection. Relax and concentrate on calm sensations. Do this exercise twice.

2. Finding Your Calm Erection

This time, when you have calmly touched your genitals for more than five minutes, decide to very slowly obtain an erection by continuing your total body relaxation, keeping your PM relaxed, and fingering your penis. Calmly let an erection happen. Patiently touch and gently pleasure your penis. The more relaxed and focused you are on the sensation, the easier it will become erect. You are practicing getting an erection with self-entrancement arousal—maximum body relaxation, minimal touch, and absence of sexual fantasy.

Be patient. Typically, it will take a number of minutes before an erection begins. Do not press it or you will undermine your physical relaxation foundation. After several minutes of consistently calm touch, increase the stimulation just a little, then be patient. You are trying to find the minimum of touch you require to get an erection. This may take some practice and patience, and may not occur the first time you do this exercise. If it does occur, be sure you are not rushing it, because you would probably conclude that you need more stimulation than is really necessary.

If an erection does not occur, keep your PM relaxed and gradually increase the touch to your penis. Try gently using both hands. Focus on the pleasure; be patient. If after three exercises you have not begun to find your calm erection, then you may begin to add mildly arousing partner interaction fantasy. Using your arousal continuum, imagine very low-arousal items (10, 12, 15, or 20). You are searching for the mildest physical and cognitive arousals that you need for an easy erection. If you come to focus on items above 25 on your arousal continuum and have not begun an easy erection, it likely means that you are not as physically relaxed as you believe. Back up and focus again on sensual relaxation.

When your calm erection begins, enjoy it for several minutes. Stay focused and be sure your PM is relaxed. Then choose to let your erection subside by stopping the touch to your penis. Do this exercise a minimum of two times.

3. Choosing to Wax and Wane

This time, choose to let your erection subside about 50 percent by stopping or changing the touch to your penis. Concentrate on the sensations. As you feel it subside, stay focused on the sensations. Then simply change the touch to gradually bring back a relaxed erection. Notice that when you're physically relaxed, it is easier to get an erection, although it may take a little more time. Notice that you can lose your erection and regain it easily when you are calm and patient.

Phase Two: Pleasure Toleration

Now that you've expanded your comfort with your body and your partner and learned relaxation and self-entrancement arousal, you're ready to expand your pleasure as a couple by learning arousal toleration together. You'll learn to better identify and respect your point of ejaculatory inevitability while tolerating progressively heightened stimulation.

Step Six: Relaxed Couple Pleasuring

Goal: Enjoy relaxed, nonerotic, sensual touch

Mark and Lisa found that the soothing, relaxing touch in this exercise helped them to explore the sensations in their bodies, increase pleasure, and overcome the barriers impeding the relaxed flow of healthy sexual response. This exercise will help you learn that when you're relaxed, touch can be very pleasant without being sexually arousing.

COUPLE EXERCISE:
RELAXED PLEASURING

Set aside one hour, and choose a private, softly lit, and comfortable place. Undress and prepare yourself to be relaxed and focused. For fifteen minutes, pleasure the entire back of your partner's nude body; then for fifteen minutes, pleasure the front of her body with the exception of her breasts and genitals. Then have her reciprocate, spending fifteen minutes on your back, then fifteen minutes on your

front, again avoiding the area around your nipples and your genitals. This touch is not intended as massage (designed to loosen up
tight muscles) but a relaxed, comforting, sensual touch, a surface
gliding, a pleasuring.

Keep your attention on your body, focusing upon the sensations you feel as you are being touched or are touching. Feel free to
guide your partner by giving verbal directions ("Your rubbing
makes me feel warm and secure," "I really like what you are doing
now," "Your kisses on my shoulder are so soothing") or taking his or
her hand, showing how you want to be touched. If your partner
caresses you in a manner that does not please you, take responsibility to speak up. Instead of complaining, you might say, "It feels
better when you press more gently," or "I would enjoy a softer
touch." Otherwise, let the time be fairly quiet so that you can concentrate on the sensations and pleasurable feelings. If your body
responds with an erection, you probably are overdoing the touch or
coming too close to erotic zones, so make subtle adjustments. If you
are relaxing with the pleasure, you will not feel sexually aroused or
erect. If you do arouse, simply focus more carefully on the pleasurable sensations, and your excitement will subside.

Feel free to experiment with sensations. Touch, hold, kiss, lick,
suck, or otherwise caress your partner's body in a way that is pleasant and interesting. You may want to explore the joy of touch by
using massage oil or talcum powder, or caressing with feathers, silk,
fleece, or flannel. Remember those little places: eyelids, toes, scalp,
behind the knees, bridge of the nose.

While you are receiving, selfishly soak up every sensation.
Enjoy your here-and-now experience, focusing on sensory pleasures.
By taking turns, you have the opportunity to concentrate on your
own feelings whether giving or receiving. Although pleasing your
partner is an important part of a sensual encounter, pleasing yourself
is equally important.

Finally, do not use the exercise as an introduction to sex. Not
having sex for at least three hours afterward will help protect the
relaxing nature of this exercise. If your mind and body anticipate
that you will have sex at the end of the exercise, this will become a
distraction from your focus on the pleasure. Remember, this is a
sensual relaxation exercise.

When you and your partner are both able to comfortably relax,
focus on the sensual pleasure, limit mental distractions to less that 20
percent of the time, and not experience erotic response (such as
erection), you are ready to move on to the next step.

Mark and Lisa did four sessions of this relaxed pleasuring exercise. At first, Mark would get an erection by simply pleasuring Lisa's legs, thighs, or stomach. Dr. Hernandez suggested that Mark focus more carefully on what he was feeling in his fingers as he touched Lisa, narrow his concentration and avoid fantasizing when looking at Lisa's breasts or genitals, and allow his body to relax. Over time, Mark was able to relax and focus more comfortably without having erections. This was an indication that he had achieved the level of comfort and relaxation needed at this step.

Step Seven: Partner Genital Exploration

Goal: Learn more about your own sensations and your partner's; enjoy calm, relaxed touch and physical relaxation in an otherwise erotic situation

In this exercise, you and your partner will take turns leading each other in an exploration of your genitals. The purpose is to provide a sensual exploration of the body's erotic parts, to practice sexual leadership with your own body, and to become more comfortable looking at and touching each other's genitals in a relaxing, nonarousing way. This exercise is a show-and-tell about your body and erogenous zones.

COUPLE EXERCISE: PARTNER GENITAL EXPLORATION

This entire exercise should take approximately one hour. Begin with thirty minutes (fifteen minutes for each of you) of relaxed pleasuring of the nongenital parts of the body. (This is a shortened version of the relaxed couple pleasuring exercise.)

Have your partner comfortably position herself in a reclining position, her back propped up with pillows. Position yourself comfortably alongside her, facing her. For the next fifteen minutes, have her lead you in an exploration of the erogenous parts of her body.

Discuss the sensations: what she prefers, what is uncomfortable. Be sure to discuss how you can enrich her pleasure. Ask questions of each other to learn or confirm what you experience. Use a scale of 1 to 10 to talk about how erotically sensitive a particular area is when relaxed.

Gently explore the sensations of her breasts, nipples, stomach and abdomen, hips and upper thighs, inner thighs, outer lips of the vagina and perineum (the area between her vagina and anus), and inside the vagina. Some women have uncomfortable feelings about examinations, associating this with impersonal gynecological exams, so let her take the lead. Be sure she feels comfortable and in control. Give her your hand and ask her to direct your touch. She might have you form a Y-shape with your index and middle fingers and show you how to gently pleasure the outer lips of her vagina. Talk, describe, and discuss.

When you are ready to explore sensations inside her vagina, have her guide you in inserting one of your fingers (usually the middle finger) and direct you in slowly pleasuring the inside of her vagina. Imagine the vagina as the face of a clock, with the top being 12:00. Have her guide your pleasuring, explaining her sensations. Many women notice they feel very little beyond three-quarters to one inch inside. Proceed around the face of the clock to 3:00, 6:00, and 9:00, stopping at each point, exploring and discussing the sensations. Work cooperatively to learn, confirm, relax, and enjoy.

Now it is your turn. Take the lead in the exploration of your body. Begin with your chest and nipples. Take your partner's hand and direct her, explaining your sensations and using the 1-to-10 scale to note the level of sensitivity you feel. Be sure you feel comfortable and in control, especially when she is exploring your testicles and penis. You might have her cup one or both testicles and describe for her your sensations, or ask her to explore different parts with her index finger, showing her how to pleasure you. Many women have heard that men's testicles are very delicate. Be sure to teach her about your testicles so she is not over- or undersensitive to you. Then explore the sensations in your penis. Have her gently place your penis back onto your stomach. Ask her to take her index finger and, beginning at the base of your penis, very slowly explore sensations up the penile shaft. Show her the more sensitive part on your penis. Be sure to give her feedback about what you are feeling each step of the way. Have her ask you questions about your sensations.

Do this exercise a minimum of three times before moving to the next step. The repetition will increase your comfort. Conscious relaxation and focus on the sensations will allow you to feel calm, pleased, and comfortable while doing what would otherwise be erotic.

Lisa and Mark engaged in the partner genital exploration exercise four times. Both were surprised that there was little erotic feeling in the genitals while in a relaxed state. By the fourth session, Mark and Lisa rated the sensations in nipples, lips of the vagina, clitoris, shaft of the penis, and even the head of the penis in the range of 1 to 3. This was quite a change from what they expected and from what occurred the first time they tried the exercise. During the first two sessions, Mark began to get an erection as Lisa guided his finger ever so slowly to different points on her breast and nipple. He had to take several deep breaths to calm himself, pause for a moment to let his erection go away, and then focus carefully on the feeling in his fingers and her explanation of the sensation. He found it difficult at first to not get an erotic movie going in his imagination, and this, he observed later, was what caused his erection. In short, he had to refrain from partner interaction arousal.

Mark and Lisa became more comfortable each time they completed this exercise, and they were surprised at how relaxed they felt in a potentially erotic situation. In fact, Mark worried that he would lose his natural excitement with Lisa's body and would have trouble getting an erection with her. Dr. Hernandez reassured Mark that now that he knew how to relax and maintain focus on his sensations, his erections would come and go easily.

Step Eight: Individual Pacing Training

Goal: During self-pleasuring, learn to become highly aroused without ejaculating by first pausing, then slowing your physical and mental stimulation

The stop-start technique, originally described by Semans (1956), is one of the skills that is most often associated with success at learning ejaculatory control. Remember the plateau phase of the sexual response cycle, which we explained in chapter 2? Stop-start pacing teaches you how to remain in the plateau phase for as long as you choose without going on to orgasm. This technique blends behavioral pacing (varying levels of physical stimulation) with cognitive pacing (choosing a more or less arousing focus for your thoughts). You learn to control your cognitive arousal by shifting between self-entrancement arousal and partner interaction arousal (in the form of fantasy).

INDIVIDUAL EXERCISE: STOP-START PACING

There are four stages of the stop-start training. Practice each stage at least three times before moving on to the next stage. This is a thirty-minute exercise, including fifteen minutes of general relaxation followed by fifteen minutes of pleasuring your penis. The approach varies according to the stage you are working on. First you pause, then you simply slow the stimulation. Then you will add fantasy (partner interaction arousal) to the mix.

The first half of the exercise is the same for all stages. Take a few moments to get comfortable on your bed, and then spend fifteen minutes gently and slowly touching and soothing your body all over with the exception of your genitals. Use this time to focus on your body's sensations and calm yourself. From time to time during this self-pleasuring, turn your attention to your PM. Tighten and relax it several times to heighten your awareness of its level of relaxation. Consciously direct your PM to relax.

1. Stimulation Pausing

In this stage, you practice using only self-entrancement arousal and preventing ejaculatory inevitability by stopping stimulation.

After the fifteen minutes of relaxing touch and PM relaxation, calmly shift your attention to your genitals. With a dry hand (no lotion or other lubrication), masturbate for fifteen minutes without ejaculation. Focus on your penis, attending to the pleasure, the sensation. The first time you do this exercise, touch very calmly, very slowly: a sensual fingering of your penis and testicles, groin, thighs. At subsequent sessions, gradually increase your touching, stroking and allowing yourself to become more excited. Do not rush. Do not push it. Do not get carried away. Keep your attention only on the sensations in your penis (no fantasy or distractions).

Eventually you will become more excited and feel that you are approaching the point of ejaculatory inevitability. When you sense this coming, stop the stimulation, hold your penis gently, and do nothing but focus on the sensation in your penis. The urge to ejaculate will subside in fifteen seconds to three minutes. You may also experience a partial loss of erection; this is common and nothing to be concerned about. When the desire to ejaculate has passed, slowly resume your masturbation. You will probably have to stop a number of times to avoid ejaculation when you first do this exercise. Keep your PM relaxed. Over time, you will learn how to recognize approaching ejaculatory inevitability, how to anticipate the need to stop, when to stop, and how long to wait. The number of times you need to stop will gradually decrease.

Here are some problems you may have:

- *You ejaculate with surprise.* When this happens, usually you are not focusing carefully on the sensations in your penis, your PM is not as relaxed as you thought, or you are trying too hard. Simply relax, play it safe (don't go too close to the brink), and focus on the physical pleasure.

- *You find you need to stop again as soon as you resume masturbating.* This means that you are not allowing sufficient time for the ejaculatory urge to diminish. Double the time you pause.

- *You get discouraged and don't think you are making any progress because you continue to ejaculate before you choose or the number of required pauses does not diminish.* This may mean that you are too tense while doing the exercise. Calm your body while you pleasure yourself. Be sure to monitor your PM. Be patient.

When you feel confident of your ability to relax your body and feel in control, and when you need only two or three stops during the fifteen minutes, you can move on.

2. Stimulation Pacing

In this stage, you continue to use only self-entrancement arousal, and this time you prevent ejaculatory inevitability by pacing (slowing, not stopping) stimulation.

After the fifteen minutes of relaxing touch and PM relaxation, masturbate for fifteen minutes without ejaculating and without stopping or pausing. When you reach high levels of excitement, make changes in your stimulation to decrease the arousal. You can slow down the pace, change the pressure you are applying, vary the site of maximum stimulation (for example, by stimulating only the shaft of your penis rather than the tip), or change the type of stroking (for example, using longer strokes or circular motions). Focus only on your body; no fantasy! Remember to relax your PM and keep it relaxed.

Find what works best for you to pace your arousal. Explore and master this. With pacing rather than stopping, more subtle types of adjustment need to be made a bit sooner. Do not hesitate to slow early. If you make the change too late, you can always stop to prevent ejaculation.

When you feel that you are doing well enough with this stage, and you're not having to stop or pause, move on to stage 3.

3. Fantasy and Stimulation Pausing

This stage begins to incorporate partner interaction arousal. You back off from the point of ejaculatory inevitability by stopping stimulation.

During the fifteen minutes of self-pleasuring, begin to fantasize about having sex with your partner. The idea is to move the focus of your concentration back and forth from your own body (self-entrancement arousal) to a fantasy of your partner (partner interaction). Spend five to fifteen seconds on your sensations, then five to fifteen seconds on the fantasy, then five seconds relaxing your PM. Start the fantasy with the first touch or kiss, and go through the stages that might occur in this imagined sexual event. You can use the sexual arousal continuum you outlined earlier.

Take your time with the imagery! You don't have to get through an entire sexual event in one session. Go slowly, calmly. Use the stop-start technique, and when you stop, imagine pausing during your fantasy sexual interaction with your lover. Imagine she is stroking you, orally pleasuring you, or having intercourse, and picture placing your hand on her hand to pause, wait, then resume. You are mentally rehearsing the stop-start technique in preparation for intercourse. Remember to keep your PM relaxed.

As you get better at this, try including in your fantasy component the erotic images you find most stimulating: imagine your penis entering her vagina, and imagine vigorous thrusting during intercourse.

Don't get discouraged if your progress is slow. This is the more challenging stage. You're learning to balance your focus on your own physical sensations, your PM, and your fantasy—all while monitoring how excited you are becoming. If you feel frustrated, simply stop or pause sooner.

When you are comfortable and in control while fantasizing erotic scenes, you are ready to move to stage 4.

4. Fantasy and Stimulation Pacing

This stage is identical to stage 3 except that now you pace (slow) rather than pause. As you make adjustments in your masturbation, imagine yourself making them in partner sex. Take it as slowly as you need to. When this stage is going well, use a lubricant on your penis to simulate the sensations of intercourse.

When you are comfortable with your individual ejaculatory control, blending self-entrancement, partner interaction fantasy, and PM relaxation, you are ready to learn couple stop-start pacing.

Step Nine: Couple Pacing Training

Goal: Learn to become highly aroused without ejaculating when your partner is stimulating you

This is the teasing-can-be-fun step! This exercise teaches you to integrate self-entrancement arousal, partner interaction arousal, and PM relaxation while your partner is pleasuring you. This is where you need your partner's assistance and patience.

COUPLE EXERCISE:
STOP-START PACING

Couple stop-start pacing consists of four stages, just like individual stop-start pacing. Each practice session takes one hour. Repeat each step until you are relaxed doing it before moving on to the next.

Each session begins with thirty minutes of relaxed couple pleasuring, which you learned in step six. Then, for fifteen minutes, your partner directs you in pleasuring her body in whatever fashion she wishes, allowing her to become highly aroused but without going on to orgasm. The final fifteen minutes is different for each of the four stages. As you work through these stages, be sure to communicate with your partner and keep your PM relaxed. All of the suggestions for individual stop-start pacing apply here as well.

1. Pausing

During your fifteen minutes of arousal practice, guide your partner to touch your penis and testicles, groin, and thighs calmly and gently. Keep your attention only on the sensations in your penis (that is, focus on self-entrancement arousal). When you feel that you are approaching the point of ejaculatory inevitability, signal her to stop stroking, pause, and gently hold your penis. Focus on the sensation as she holds you. When the desire to ejaculate has passed, slowly resume stimulation.

2. Pacing

Instead of stopping or pausing to prevent ejaculation, work with your partner to slow the stroking without stopping. Then have her increase stimulation again when you are relaxed and not at risk of ejaculating. Be sure to focus only on your sensations, not on your partner. Remember that you can always stop to prevent ejaculation.

3. Pausing with Partner Focus

Gradually shift the focus of your concentration from your own sensations to enjoyment of your partner (looking at her or watching her touch you) to relaxing your PM. When you first shift your focus to your partner, be careful not to overstimulate yourself—remember your arousal continuum. When you realize you are getting close to ejaculatory inevitability, pause. As you progress, you may want to use a lubricant on your penis to heighten the pleasure and more closely simulate feelings of intercourse. You are training yourself to enjoy more pleasure without ejaculating.

4. Pacing with Partner Focus

This final stage builds on stage 3 by slowing instead of pausing.

You are well on your way to learning to integrate relaxation, cooperation, self-entrancement arousal, and partner interaction arousal. You gain significant power by learning to control the pacing of your arousal.

Mark and Lisa found that during the fifteen minutes Mark was pleasuring Lisa, he had to focus carefully on the touch he was giving, on the physical sensation in his hand, and close his mind to Lisa's sounds and movement—in short, he had to not watch the erotic movie he was facilitating. At first, when Lisa was pleasuring Mark, he needed to pause often, but by the third session he could arouse close to ejaculation, keep his PM relaxed, and enjoy the pleasure of high arousal without ejaculating.

The key features of Mark's work during this step were relaxing the PM, focusing principally on sensual self-entrancement arousal and then carefully beginning to allow some partner interaction focus, and pacing the touch he received from Lisa. Monitoring these three features was quite complicated at first—he felt like he was juggling too many things—but with repetition and his just-be-good-enough attitude, it became easier and more comfortable.

Mark became concerned when he ejaculated during the second exercise (pacing without partner focus). He was feeling relaxed, enjoying the feel of Lisa stroking his penis, concentrating on the pleasurable sensations, monitoring his PM to keep it relaxed, and anticipating the point of inevitability—and yet he still ejaculated. When he later evaluated what happened, it became clear that while he was doing all the right things, he still was allowing an erotic movie to play out in his mind. Mark realized that even though he was carefully orchestrating his focus, he was also having brief images of partner interaction. He looked at Lisa stroking him, glimpsed her breasts, her eyes, even had images of intercourse flash through his mind. When he realized this, it made sense that he had lost control and subsequently ejaculated. He was amazed to experience this power of his mind. By adjusting his mental focus, he could regulate his arousal. It was a dramatic demonstration to Mark of the difference between self-entrancement and partner interaction arousal. This was one of his most important experiences in learning to pace his sexual arousal.

Phase Three: Pleasure Saturation

In this phase, you'll learn to experience prolonged intercourse and enjoy more intense sexual stimulation without ejaculating quickly. You'll learn to stay relaxed while welcoming the sensual pleasure of intercourse. Pleasure saturation—soaking yourselves with pleasure—is one of your rewards for learning ejaculatory control. We'll coach you as you integrate or orchestrate the skills to overcome PE during intercourse. At first this might be awkward, but with practice it will become second nature.

Step Ten: Intimate Intercourse

Goal: Learn to calmly adapt to intercourse

Mark and Lisa gained confidence from their success with stop-start pacing, but both felt anxious about this next step. Intercourse was where Mark had the most trouble controlling his arousal and ejaculation. Their anxiety was understandable. Many men with PE feel that intercourse is the ultimate test of their success in ejaculatory control.

This exercise will help you take the next step successfully by showing you how to keep your PM relaxed during insertion and by teaching you to stay relaxed while *acclimating* (adjusting) to the sensation of your partner's vagina.

COUPLE EXERCISE: INITIATING AND ACCLIMATING TO INTERCOURSE

Relax by doing thirty minutes of couple relaxed pleasuring. Then lie on your back as your partner straddles you and helps you gain an erection. Using only self-entrancement arousal (that is, focusing on your own sensations), allow yourself to become aroused and erect. When you are ready to begin intercourse, be sure your PM is relaxed at the 2 or 3 level. This is particularly important at the moment of starting intercourse because when she is inserting your penis, it is natural for the PM to tighten or "salute" as a reflex. If you allow this to happen, you are unwittingly tightening the very muscles involved in ejaculation, thereby "priming the pump." Relaxing the PM muscle, especially during insertion, will offer some reserve.

While focusing on your penis, keep the PM relaxed while your partner slowly inserts you. Once inside, simply rest, enjoying the warmth and closeness. Focus on the pleasure in your penis. Wait, calmly expecting to reach the physical pleasure "saturation point" where your penis acclimates to the warmth and sensuousness of her vagina. For most men, this sensation develops after approximately ten to fifteen minutes of resting inside the vagina, but we have seen a range of seven to twenty-seven minutes. Move only minimally to maintain your erection. Your objective is to remain entirely passive, alternating your attention between maintaining PM relaxation and focusing on the pleasure in your penis. It is important to focus on self-entrancement arousal throughout this step.

After acclimation occurs, you can begin to tolerate and enjoy more intense pleasure while you maintain ejaculatory control. Enjoy at least fifteen minutes of relaxed intercourse, then feel free to choose to ejaculate. Rest for a moment to catch your breath, then stay with your partner and pleasure her in whatever ways she prefers. She is also now free to experience orgasm if she wishes.

When Mark and Lisa first tried this, it took Mark eighteen minutes of relaxed intercourse to begin to experience acclimation. The sensation of acclimating is commonly vague at first, so we recommend that you wait three minutes beyond when you think it is happening, just to play it safe. The good news is that once you experience acclimation, it usually does not take as long in future sessions, but at first ten, fifteen, or twenty minutes or longer is not unusual. In successive sessions, Mark's acclimating time lessened to about eight minutes.

When the acclimation was established, he and Lisa began to slowly move during intercourse. Mark maintained his focus on the sensations of relaxed pleasure. At first he feared this would make him ejaculate, and he was surprised to find it actually helped him not to. Mark could accept the pleasure without moving to the point of ejaculatory inevitability. They could pause or pace movement to avoid ejaculation. Both were amazed that they were able to have twenty minutes or more of careful intercourse after acclimating (for a total of more than thirty minutes of intercourse), even though it was reserved and subdued. Lisa said she loved the relaxed feeling of closeness while calmly enjoying intercourse.

As Mark's comfort increased, he was able to keep his PM at a 2 or 3 ranking as he focused on the pleasure in his penis. So Dr. Hernandez suggested that Mark cautiously begin adding moments of partner involvement arousal, focusing on Lisa's body and movements and even looking into Lisa's eyes. After some shyness, they both remarked how much they liked this. They were surprised that this also felt calming and close.

Step Eleven: Progressive Intercourse

Goal: Integrate the skills and become open to spontaneity

Buoyed by their progress with the acclimating step, Mark and Lisa decided they were ready to put together everything they'd learned by trying *progressive intercourse*. They took thirty minutes at the start of a session to enjoy pleasant, soothing touch. They talked little, focusing on the pleasing sensations. At first they simply enjoyed relaxed intercourse, waiting for the acclimating. When this occurred, they began to enjoy slow, reserved intercourse movement for ten minutes or so. At first only Lisa would do the moving (to help Mark focus on relaxed pleasure), but gradually Mark and Lisa would take turns moving, then move together cooperatively and slowly.

Mark had some trouble keeping himself focused, but gradually got into a pattern of alternately focusing on the pleasure in his penis for fifteen seconds and monitoring his PM for five to ten seconds to keep it relaxed.

When he became comfortable with this pattern, they switched from Lisa on top to Mark on top. This required more careful management of PM relaxation because being on top uses the muscles differently and makes it harder to relax them. Mark also had to be more careful to stay focused on sensations in his own body. When this, too, became easier, he began to add small doses of a third focus: Lisa! Mark allowed himself five-second increments of partner interaction arousal (looking at Lisa's body) before returning his attention to the sensation in his penis, the PM, and his penis again.

Orchestrating this was taxing at first, but it worked because their intercourse movement was slow. Mark was doing okay pacing and didn't need to pause now. Slowly Mark became more comfortable and confident integrating PM relaxation, exquisite focus on the pleasure in his penis, and calm and gradual inclusion of partner interaction arousal.

During the fourth practice session of progressive intercourse, Mark inadvertently ejaculated. His first emotional reaction was to feel deeply despondent, but he was wonderfully helped by Lisa's gentle reminder that he was making such good progress. He also realized his reaction was the same old negative one—feeling like a failure. He caught himself and emotionally regrouped. He realized that Lisa was correct: it was just a goof, not a relapse. He *was* making good progress.

From this setback, Mark learned that he needed to guarantee that acclimation had occurred by waiting an extra minute, and needed to not get sloppy about maintaining his focus on self-entrancement arousal, monitoring his PM, and being careful about the partner interaction arousal. This is where the arousal continuum he had designed earlier was helpful. When he evaluated what happened when he ejaculated without choosing to, he realized that he was not only focusing less on his body and the PM, but also focusing more on Lisa's body and movements. Mark recognized that he had made a mental mistake: he had shifted too quickly from a moderately arousing item on his continuum (a 55 item, "watching her breasts as she moved up and down on me") to a highly arousing item (a 90 item, "imagining Lisa getting close to orgasm"). This confirmed for Mark the power of cognitive pacing.

Mark was able to accept more and more stimulation as he balanced focus on the pleasure in his penis (self-entrancement), PM relaxation, Lisa's body and activity (partner interaction), and at times imaginary items on his arousal continuum that were less exciting than the actual activity he and Lisa were sharing. Here he was coordinating four cognitive and behavioral pacing techniques, grounded in physiological relaxation, within a cooperative relationship and with the pause technique as a backup.

As Mark became more proficient—and more confident—he and Lisa began to focus more on her feeling freer to do what she desired. They had more sessions where Mark asked her to have intercourse her way—a kind of teasing with intercourse similar to the stop-start teasing with manual stimulation. This allowed Lisa to loosen the restraints she had felt for so long, and allowed Mark to practice his cognitive pacing techniques. As Mark and Lisa cooperated more, they increased their comfort, pleasure, and confidence. They were focusing more on pleasure and closeness and less on ejaculation.

It was not all easy, however. There were good days and not-so-good days. It took longer than they had wished. There were moments of worry, sessions that bombed. They had to remind each other what they were trying to do with each step so that they did not revert to old ways of thinking, feeling, and acting. It took self-discipline and cooperation. But they cooperated. They concentrated. Their alliance and patience were indispensable. They were good enough. They were feeling closer, warmer, more secure together. They were succeeding.

COUPLE EXERCISE: PROGRESSIVE INTERCOURSE

You are ready to experience more variety, excitement, and pleasure during intercourse. Follow Mark and Lisa's example. Remember to establish intercourse acclimation and to balance your focus for adequate management of arousal, but also allow yourself to enjoy expanding your freedom with intercourse.

As you add partner interaction arousal, keep in mind your arousal continuum. Don't drag race. That is, don't start at 50! Begin slowly, gradually, gently. Stay focused on each specific activity or image for at least fifteen seconds before changing. Shift attention in small steps. Do not change from one focus to another that is more than five points above.

If you have a setback, simply learn from it and regroup. Remember, you are still learning to integrate the different dimensions of arousal management. With practice, you will find coordinating your arousal becomes second nature, requiring less conscious attention. This reopens your sexual relationship to more personal feelings and deeper intimacy. Enjoy!

What If These Skills Don't Work for You?

While this program is helpful for most men and couples, do not be discouraged if some of the skills do not work as well for you. It is not well understood why the same skills that help many men don't work for others—or may even have the opposite effect. For example, some men find that PM relaxation does not help. Rather, these men find that tightening, holding, and exhausting the PM is more effective. So don't be afraid to experiment with how various techniques work for your body. If you get stuck, it would be wise to consult with an experienced marital and sex therapist to help you develop your own way to integrate the skills for increasing ejaculatory control and sexual intimacy.

9

Couple Sexuality: Building an Intimate, Interactive Couple Sexual Style

Now that you've built solid skills to improve your sexual relationship, you'll want to consider how this fits into the "big picture" of your relationship. Your relationship has undoubtedly changed as you've learned the skills in this book. You've developed new levels of intimacy, communication, and closeness. This is a good time to ask yourself what you want your relationship to be like, and how sexuality will fit in.

You owe it to yourself and your partner to develop a comfortable, pleasurable, and functional couple sexual style. This will help you maintain the progress you've made in dealing with PE and will strengthen your long-term sexual and relationship satisfaction. Healthy sexuality is a team effort, not an individual performance. Emotional and sexual intimacy is the glue of your couple bond. Your intimate relationship is the energy source for a vital, satisfying sexuality.

The traditional belief was that the more emotional intimacy, the better the marriage. In fact, that is a myth. A crucial factor in developing a cooperative marital style is maintaining balance between autonomy and intimacy; that is, balance between individuality and couple focus.

In this chapter, we'll take a look at the common marital styles and the role sexuality plays in each. We will examine both strengths and potential problems of each marital and sexual style. We will also examine dating and serious relationships and the role of sexuality in these. Finally, we'll guide you through actively and consciously choosing a couple style that works for you.

Marital and Sexual Styles

There are four marital styles. In their order of frequency, they are *complementary, conflict minimizing, best friend,* and *emotionally expressive.* Of course, these are not pure categories, but one style commonly predominates for a given couple. Each style describes a different approach to intimacy, autonomy, communication, power dynamics, and the role of sex within the relationship, as well as a different approach to initiating sex, interacting during sex, and ending sexual encounters.

The Complementary Couple Style

The complementary couple style is the most common. The partners respect each other's contributions, each partner has his or her domain of competence and power, and each values moderate intimacy balanced by a clear sense of autonomy. These couples are able to resolve conflicts and maintain dialogue about difficult issues. Each partner feels valued, respected, and cared for. The emotional tone of the relationship is affirming.

Complementary couples have a good sexual relationship, seeing sexuality as a positive, integral component in the marriage but certainly not the most important factor.

The trap for this marital style is to fall into a pattern of routine, mechanical sex. Sex becomes a low priority, occurring late at night after all the important things in life (like putting the children to sleep, paying bills, walking the dog, and watching the *The Tonight Show*) are done. Sex might be functional (for instance, the man maintains good ejaculatory control), but it lacks excitement and emotional intimacy. The couple thinks about their premarital sexual experiences—and possibly their experience working together to learn ejaculatory control—and they miss that sense of connection and specialness.

Marital sexuality cannot rest on its past success; setting aside couple time and valuing intimate sexuality are crucial. To maintain healthy sexuality, complementary couples can decide to make sexual initiation a shared domain, or one spouse can claim it as his or her domain. Ideally, each spouse would be comfortable initiating and each would feel free to say no and perhaps offer an alternative way to connect.

Traditionally, it is the male who makes sexuality his domain. This is fine as long as he is committed to maintaining a satisfying sexuality. The danger is that he might overemphasize intercourse as a performance at the expense of intimacy, affection, and pleasuring. Improved ejaculatory control alone will not be enough to ensure the woman's anticipation, pleasure, and satisfaction. The other danger, especially with the aging of the people and the marriage, is that the man's focus on performance and intercourse subverts satisfaction. A broad-based, variable, flexible approach to couple sexuality is more likely to promote desire and satisfaction, and helps inoculate the couple against sexual dysfunction. Maintaining a vital sexual relationship is a couple task, with the woman's sexual feelings and "voice" playing an integral role.

The Conflict-Minimizing Couple Style

The conflict-minimizing couple style is the most stable. These marriages are usually organized along traditional gender roles, with the man as the prime income generator and the woman the homemaker, although other patterns are common in recent years. They are characterized by avoidance of strong emotional expression (especially anger), limited intimacy, and emphasis on children, family, and religious values. The emotional and practical rules of the marriage are clearly understood and consistently implemented. Conflict-minimizing couples value security over intimacy and family over the couple relationship. People value this marital style because of the predictability and security.

The role of sex is de-emphasized. Often, the limited emotional expression in these relationships results in inhibited erotic expression. Sexual problems are typically minimized. The couple avoids confronting sexual issues.

Initiating sex and establishing sexual frequency is viewed as the man's role. The sexual scenario emphasizes intercourse, with a focus on one-way foreplay rather than mutual pleasuring. The expectation is that she will function like him: have a single orgasm during intercourse. Sex is his domain, affection and feelings are her domain.

There are several possible sexual traps with this marital style. The biggest is that sex becomes marginal and mechanical, and eventually very infrequent. The couple falls into the cycle of a low-sex or no-sex marriage. Another trap is that the focus on intercourse makes the man vulnerable to erectile dysfunction and inhibited sexual desire as he ages. When couples stop having sex, whether at forty, sixty, or eighty, it is almost always the man's unilateral, unspoken decision. He is too frustrated and embarrassed by sexual problems and decides sex is not worth the effort. The partners have not been intimate friends, which makes it hard to develop intimate, interactive sexuality.

Conflict-minimizing couples miss the opportunity to use conflicts to deepen intimacy, and underplay the positive role of sexuality in sharing pleasure and energizing their marital bond. We urge couples who choose this marital style to be sure that sexuality, including enjoying ejaculatory control and intercourse, plays a healthy 15 to 20 percent role in marital vitality and satisfaction.

The Best Friend Couple Style

The best friend couple style is characterized by the highest degree of intimacy, acceptance, and sharing; equitable distribution of roles and responsibilities; and a strong commitment to a close, vital marriage. Although this is the cultural ideal, this marital style runs the risk of leading to disappointment and alienation when emotional and sexual expectations are not met or there are irresolvable conflicts.

When both individuals choose this marital style and devote the time and psychological energy to make it successful, this can be a very impressive marriage. However, it is not the right marital style for the majority of couples. Best friend couples have a high divorce rate, based on disappointment and resentment toward the spouse and the marriage. The marriage cannot live up to the "love means never having to say you're sorry" promise.

Sex is a positive, integral, vital resource. Sexuality energizes the marital bond and makes it special. The couple enjoys touching both inside and outside the bedroom. Intimacy, pleasuring, and eroticism are valued by both people and integrated into their lovemaking. They develop a sexual style that is flexible and responsive to the feelings and preferences of both partners.

What are the traps of this marital style? The biggest emotional trap is relationship enmeshment, meaning that the couple sacrifices autonomy and individuality for the sake of the couple bond. When things do not work well, they may regress to hurt, blaming, and resentment. Disappointment and disillusion rob the marriage of vitality. The couple lacks conflict resolution skills and is bitter over thwarted hopes and expectations.

The biggest sexual trap is inhibited sexual desire. Ideally, intimacy and couple time serve as bridges to sexual desire, but too much intimacy can stifle erotic feelings. In truth, either too little or too much intimacy can subvert desire. If the couple is so emotionally close that they cannot make sexual requests, if they de-eroticize each other, or if they are so worried about hurting each other that they do not share negative sexual feelings, they are in trouble. They need to have a mutually comfortable level of intimacy that promotes connection and sexual desire.

Best friend couples are not assertive in dealing with sexual dysfunction or dissatisfaction. They expect that each should know what the other is thinking and what the other wants without having to ask or explain. The cultural myth is that love is all we need. But when there is a sexual dysfunction, love is not enough. Warm feelings and caring communication are very helpful, but are not enough to overcome PE and maintain a satisfying sexual relationship. The combination of taking personal responsibility and working as an intimate team can be a challenge for best friend couples. They often become stuck in a cycle of avoidance, not wanting to push the other, waiting for the other to initiate. Avoidance compounds the sexual problem.

The Emotionally Expressive Couple Style

The emotionally expressive couple style is the most volatile and unstable, but the most engaging, fun, and erotic. Intimacy in this style is like an accordion: sometimes very close, other times very distant. Emotionally expressive couples have the highest intensity of feelings, both loving and angry. These couples value intimacy and vitality without being afraid of conflict or anger. When this marital style works well, the couple has a vibrant and exciting relationship. They value sexuality that is spontaneous, adventuresome, playful, and energizing.

Unfortunately, this is the most unstable marital style, the most likely to result in divorce. The conflicts become too frequent and intense. Emotionally expressive couples can deal with disappointment, anger, and conflict, but if they cross the line into personal put-downs, contempt, and disrespect, this breaks the marital bond.

There are a number of potential sexual problems. A particularly unhealthy pattern is to use sex to make up after an abusive fight. It is poisonous for physical or emotional fights to serve as foreplay for sex. Another problem is that a gradual, step-by-step approach to dealing with PE or another sexual dysfunction—or a relapse—is not compatible with this couple style. They want a more spontaneous, freewheeling approach. If the sexual problem is not quickly resolved, they fall into the trap of feeling demoralized, bitter, and blaming. Problematic sex increases the risk of an affair or breakup.

To combat these traps, the emotionally expressive couple needs to remain aware of respecting personal and sexual boundaries. If there is a sexual problem or dysfunction, they must address it without putting down the spouse or destabilizing the relationship.

Choosing a Marital and Sexual Style

It is important for you and your partner to adopt a couple style, especially in how you deal with intimacy and conflicts. It is crucial that you adopt a sexual style that is compatible with, and hopefully enhances, your marital style. One style is not better than another, but mutual endorsement of your chosen couple and sexual style is part of being a marital team. It is not the man's (or the woman's) decision to make alone, but a cooperative choice based on respect and empathy for each spouse's preferences, needs, and values.

As you choose your style, the two most important issues to address are the amount of intimacy and the importance of sexuality. Intimacy includes sexuality, but is much more than sexuality. Especially important in emotional intimacy is the degree and quality of personal self-disclosure and empathy. Sexual intimacy includes affectionate, playful, sensual, and erotic touch in addition to intercourse. An example of a problematic intimacy and sexuality pattern is when one spouse (typically the woman) desires high levels of emotional intimacy, while the other spouse wants sex to be the main source of connection. This couple is likely to have a "pursuer" and a "distancer." When couples fall into the pursuer-distancer trap, both emotional intimacy and sexuality suffer. Sex ought not to become a power struggle, but a mutual, voluntary, and pleasure-oriented experience within an emotionally satisfying relationship.

Traditional sexual socialization dictates that males value sexual frequency and eroticism while females value intimacy and affection. This generates heated arguments on talk shows and in bars, but sheds little light on the reality and complexity of couple sexuality. To honestly assess your desires about your sexual relationship, you and your partner need to look beyond rigid sex roles. This may be particularly difficult for conflict-minimizing couples.

In choosing the marital and sexual style that's right for you, discuss together the strengths and vulnerabilities of each style. For example, the sexual style least impacted by PE and other sexual problems is the conflict-minimizing style. Sexual expectations are lower and sexual problems de-emphasized. Marital rules are very important for conflict-minimizing couples. Yet these couples face crises when an affair violates the core rule of fidelity or an infertility problem threatens the core value of family. So a conflict-minimizing couple may be able to take PE in stride, but may be less resilient in other ways.

Nick and Donna's Story

Before Nick and Donna started working on ejaculatory control together, Nick had given no thought to a couple or sexual style; his focus was on intercourse frequency as a way to compensate for PE. Donna had hoped for a best friend marriage with abundant communication and touching. If anything, Nick tended toward the conflict-minimizing style, and he especially did not want to talk about sexual problems. Nick's emphasis on intercourse, Donna's frustration with the chronic PE, her disappointment with his reluctance to talk about sexual issues, and her resentment at always being the one to reach out for affection upset her deeply. She questioned Nick's commitment and the viability of the marriage.

The ejaculatory control program was successful for Nick and Donna. Much to Nick's surprise, slowing down the sexual process, focusing on pleasure, taking medication (Nick had neurologic system PE), and especially learning to do a good-enough job of using the psychosexual skills dramatically improved their sexual enjoyment and satisfaction. Donna enjoyed her role as an active, involved spouse during the ejaculatory control exercises. Nick appreciated Donna as an intimate ally in facing up to and changing PE.

Nick was now willing to address general relationship issues as well as a PE relapse prevention program. Donna appreciated this, but was still bothered by Nick's reluctance to discuss emotional issues. Finally, Nick disclosed that he feared that Donna's demands for emotional intimacy were really a hidden agenda to limit his personal autonomy. He was afraid she did not so much want to be close to him as to overwhelm him emotionally and be critical of him. Donna had grown up with the cultural myth that the more intimacy, the better. Nick reassured her that he loved her and valued the marriage but did not want to lose his autonomy or feel smothered.

Contrary to gender myths, men have similar needs for intimacy and security as women. The difference is not in needs, but in fears. The man fears being controlled or being seen as deficient or failing his partner. As they discussed their feelings, preferences, and fears, it became clear to Nick and Donna that a complementary couple style would fit them best. This allowed a balance of autonomy and togetherness, with moderate amounts of emotional intimacy, and fit well with the personal responsibility–intimate team approach to sexuality.

Both Nick and Donna were highly motivated to maintain their sexual gains around ejaculatory control and sexual enjoyment and not allow a relapse. It was important to Nick that Donna realize that he was more emotionally open to her than to any other person in his life, and that he highly valued her and the marriage and enjoyed marital sexuality. At the same time, he needed to have a personal and emotional life apart from her. He especially wanted the freedom to hang out with his buddies from the soccer team, and the time and space to keep active in local politics. This was not a rejection of Donna, but something which was healthy for him. Nick was an antsy, high-energy guy who found sitting and talking about feelings uncomfortable. He and Donna developed a pattern of doing house chores in tandem and talking about emotional, sexual, and life-planning issues as they worked side by side.

Men in Dating or Living-Together Relationships

Many men with PE are single, divorced, or in cohabitating relationships. How do the couple and sexual styles relate to them? Consider that there are three levels of relationship connection: sexual friendships, lover relationships, and serious relationships. At all levels of a relationship, there are two important guidelines. The first is to treat the woman with respect and have an understanding that you will try to not do anything emotionally or sexually that is harmful to her or to yourself. The second is to be realistic about the relationship and not to overpromise or be manipulative.

A sexual friendship relationship is just what it sounds like: you are friends who have an active sexual relationship. As with any other friendship, you want to treat the person well, expect to be treated well in turn, and freely share activities and emotions. However, you do not promise a lifelong relationship or change life plans, career, or where you live for the woman, nor do you ask her to make those changes for you. Both people are direct and clear about their expectations. Whether the relationship lasts six months or three years, the reality is it will end. Hopefully, you wish each other well and remain friends, but there are no guarantees.

The lover relationship involves more closeness, more sharing (you may or may not live together), and more of an emotional investment. Lovers meet each other's families, make long-term vacation and holiday plans, and integrate each other into their lives. However, you do not change your life or career plans for a lover. You do not promise a lifetime commitment or plan to have children in a lover relationship.

The serious relationship has the potential to result in marriage. This is the type of relationship in which you consider changing your life in tandem with your partner and discuss all the hard and sensitive issues involved in sharing your lives emotionally, practically, financially, and sexually.

Issues of respect, trust, and emotional and sexual intimacy are just as relevant for nonmarried couples as for married ones. However, sexuality—including PE—should not make or break the future of the relationship. For example, the fact that the woman helped you with ejaculatory control does not mean that you owe her—or that she owes you—a lifelong commitment. Conversely, struggling with a sexual dysfunction is problematic but need not be a reason to terminate a relationship. As in a marriage, sexuality should play an important but not primary role.

Developing Your Couple Sexual Style

Your task is to establish your unique sexual style by exploring and sharing your sexual desires, feelings, and preferences. This exercise is divided into phases, the first to do individually. Then you'll share your thoughts and reach understandings and agreements about your unique couple style. You'll discover what is uniquely and mutually pleasurable and satisfying for you.

EXERCISE: DEVELOPING YOUR COUPLE SEXUAL STYLE

1. Think about and then write out (this makes it more concrete) the answers to the following questions. Do not be "politically correct" or try to second-guess your partner. Be free and explicit.

   - How much intimacy do you want in your life and relationship?

   - What are the most important emotions you want to share in your relationship?

   - What is your preferred way to deal with differences and conflicts?

   - What is your preferred couple style: complementary, conflict minimizing, best friend, or emotionally expressive?

   - How important is sex in your life? How important is your relationship?

- In terms of affectionate touch, do you prefer kissing, holding hands, or hugging?
- How much do you enjoy cuddling? How important is it to you?
- How do you distinguish affectionate touch from seductive or sensual touch?
- How much do you enjoy sensual touch? Do you prefer taking turns or mutually giving and receiving?
- What is the meaning and value of playful touching? How comfortable are you with affectionate nicknames for your genitals?
- How much do you enjoy erotic scenarios and techniques? Do you prefer single stimulation or multiple stimulation, taking turns or mutual stimulation, using external stimuli or not? Do you enjoy erotic sex as a route to orgasm or only as a pleasuring experience?
- What is your preferred intercourse position? Man on top, woman on top, rear entry, side to side? What type of thrusting do you prefer? In and out? Circular? Deep inside? Shallow? Do you want to engage in multiple stimulation during intercourse?
- How much do you value afterplay as a part of your lovemaking style?

2. Read your partner's responses and then carefully discuss together each question, clarifying both the practical and emotional dimensions. Remember that you are not clones of each other. You want to maintain your individuality and not feel embarrassed or apologetic about your emotional and sexual desires. Your preferences and sensitivities are part of who you are as a sexual person and must be integrated into your couple style for you to be truly satisfied.

3. Divide your answers into three categories:

Areas you agree on. These will enhance your enjoyment and satisfaction with each other and your relationship. For example, you both agree that you want a complementary couple style. You want sex to play a 15 to 20 percent energizing role; there are no major sexual secrets or conflicts; you both enjoy affectionate and playful touch more than sensual touch; on occasion you find erotic sex to orgasm highly satisfying; you agree on two favorite intercourse positions; and you both value quiet, bonding afterplay.

Areas you can reach agreement on. Identify differences you can accept and perhaps even enjoy. Perhaps one spouse prefers a conflict-minimizing couple style while the other wants the closeness of the complementary style; one partner values sharing daily feelings and experiences while the other is more emotionally reserved; the spouse who puts more value on sex agrees to be the prime initiator; one person prefers kissing and the other holding hands; one would rather do sexual touching standing up and the other likes lying in bed; he likes verbalizing sexual fantasies while she likes to close her eyes and fantasize; she likes to switch intercourse positions while he prefers to be on top. These are not matters of right or wrong. You can integrate your preferences or take turns. Enjoy your partner's sexual style. Remember, an involved, aroused partner is the best aphrodisiac.

Differences to accept or adapt to. Finally, when there are genuine major differences between you, work to accept or adapt to them. For example, one wants a conflict-minimizing relationship while the other wants an emotionally expressive style; one puts a very high priority on sex while the other is indifferent; one wants a daily sensual massage and the other hates massage; she wants to use a vibrator during intercourse to help her be orgasmic and he is turned off by the vibrator; he wants to try a variety of intercourse positions but she strongly prefers rear entry; he likes being sexual early in the morning while she only wants to be sexual late at night; he wants to experiment with swinging relationships and she values monogamy. It is not easy, or even possible, to integrate many of these differences, but there are two major coping strategies. One is to acknowledge your differences but not let them turn into a power struggle. Instead, accept them and try to work around them. It helps to remember that difference does not equal rejection. The second strategy is to agree to enter couple therapy to understand the meaning of the differences, and, with the help of the professional, find a common ground for intimacy and sexuality.

The goal of this exercise is to develop a comfortable, pleasurable, functional, and mutually satisfying couple sexual style. This exercise encourages you to take personal responsibility for your sexuality and to grow as a unique, intimate team.

You can be proud of yourselves for working together to address PE and improve ejaculatory control. In sharing emotional and sexual feelings and preferences, you'll increase understanding, empathy, and acceptance. This will provide the foundation for a couple sexual style that ensures both satisfaction and security.

10

Enjoying Sex and
Preventing Relapse

It took time, energy, and cooperation for you to learn ejaculatory control. You cannot rest on your laurels; you need to devote time and energy to maintain a vital sexuality and prevent relapse. To now expect that PE will never reoccur is unrealistic and sets you up for feelings of failure and sets the couple up to return to the blame-counterblame cycle. Positive, realistic expectations include accepting that arousal and orgasm are inherently variable. Whether once every ten times, once a month, or once a year, rapid ejaculation will reoccur. This is a normal part of good-enough sex. The reality is that rapid ejaculation is an occasional part of most couples' sexual experience, even invited: a "quickie." Especially important is to not panic and feel you are back to square one each time you experience rapid ejaculation. The key is to accept the occasional episode of rapid ejaculation as normal, treat it as a lapse, and commit to not allowing it to become a pattern (relapse).

In this chapter, we'll help you develop a personal, specific relapse prevention plan. It is crucial that you decide how you'll respond when PE occurs rather than hope it will magically never happen again. We'll take a look at the cognitive, behavioral, and emotional foundations of relapse prevention. We'll briefly review the key concepts from the ejaculatory control program. Then we will present ten specific strategies and techniques to promote healthy sexuality and prevent relapse. You can choose two to four strategies that are relevant to you and incorporate them in your couple sexual style.

The Foundation of Relapse Prevention

You've already formed the basis for relapse prevention by developing a comprehensive understanding of PE, identifying all the factors contributing to your PE, using all your resources, learning a range of steps and skills, following the personal responsibility–intimate team model of change, and building a couple sexual style that integrates intimacy, pleasuring, and eroticism and emphasizes realistic expectations of ejaculatory control and couple sex.

You can think of relapse prevention in terms of its cognitive, behavioral, and emotional foundations.

The Cognitive Foundation of Relapse Prevention

The most important cognitive approach to preventing relapse is to accept that on occasion you will ejaculate rapidly. Treat these experiences as a normal variation, not a cue for anticipatory or performance anxiety. This allows you (and your partner) to think of the experience as a lapse but not be afraid of a relapse. Cognitively, you can approach the next encounter with positive anticipation, relaxing more, using more self-entrancement arousal, enjoying a pleasurable buildup of stimulation, perhaps purposely using slow-down or stop-start pacing, and inviting your partner to control the type and speed of intercourse thrusting.

A key to relapse prevention is shifting your focus from performance-oriented intercourse to involvement in the whole lovemaking process, affection through afterplay. Intercourse is the natural extension of intimacy, pleasuring, and eroticism. It is a continuation of the pleasuring process, not a pass-fail test apart from this. Decide to let the length of intercourse vary with your desires. The skills you have learned will aid you in maintaining reasonable control over when you choose to ejaculate. Keep the perspective that you are sharing with your partner, not performing for her.

Think of your partner as your intimate friend whose pleasure and arousal feed yours rather than as a demanding critic for whom you must perform. Welcome her arousal, especially during intercourse, rather than feeling intimidated that she has to hold back so you do not ejaculate. Enjoy both her arousal and your own. Enjoy your orgasm as well as her orgasm; orgasm need not occur in perfect sequence for it to be satisfying.

Our concept of good-enough ejaculatory control and a good-enough sexual relationship is crucial for relapse prevention. Decide that your goal is to be good enough, not perfect.

The Behavioral Foundation of Relapse Prevention

The most important behavioral foundation for relapse prevention is to generalize your comfort and confidence with stop-start and arousal pacing techniques. You learned these skills in a systematic manner in the ejaculatory control exercises; now the challenge is to use them in unstructured, spontaneous sex to maintain good-enough ejaculatory control. You'll need to integrate these techniques into your couple sexual style. If there has been a break in your regular rhythm of sexual intercourse (if one of you has been traveling or has been ill), you may find it helpful to briefly return to using the techniques in a more structured way.

You want to aim for sexual encounters that involve a relaxed sexual pace (not drag racing); giving and receiving pleasure-oriented touching; being comfortable with the plateau phase and maintaining arousal; transitioning to intercourse as a continuation of the pleasuring process; monitoring your PM, using intercourse acclimation if needed; varying intercourse movements (such as using circular or longer strokes) at moderate levels of speed; moving to orgasm as a natural extension of the erotic flow; enjoying the orgasmic experience physically, emotionally, and relationally; and being an active participant in the afterplay phase.

Ejaculatory control requires a regular rhythm of sexual experiences with both people being involved and valuing their sexual relationship. The risk is regressing to infrequent, low-quality sex, which promotes a return to PE.

The Emotional Foundation of Relapse Prevention

Interpersonally, an important relapse prevention approach is to value and reinforce your couple sexual style and to view each other as intimate friends. Your feelings for each other are the glue that bonds you. Personal responsibility for sexuality, emotional sharing, and being an intimate team are ongoing parts of your life and relationship. Especially important is setting aside quality couple time when you share feelings and are empathic about your life and relationship, including your sexuality. You want to enjoy a broad-based, flexible couple style that integrates emotional intimacy, pleasuring, and eroticism.

Key Concepts in Ejaculatory Control

As you develop your couple sexual style and work to maintain ejaculatory control, you'll want to keep in mind the key concepts you've learned. Consider which concepts were the most difficult for you to master. These are the ones that will need your continued attention in order to prevent relapse.

- Premature ejaculation is the most frequent male sexual problem. The majority of adolescents and young adults begin as rapid ejaculators. Thirty percent of adult males complain of quick ejaculation.

- Realistic expectations and goals are crucial. Base them on the physical realities of your body, accurate knowledge, and the principle of just being good enough.

- Do-it-yourself techniques to reduce arousal do not help in gaining ejaculatory control. By interfering with arousal, these techniques can cause erectile dysfunction.

- The strategy for ejaculatory control is counterintuitive. Rather than decreasing pleasure, you want to increase comfort, awareness, and pleasure.

- The important individual skills for ejaculatory control are physical relaxation during lovemaking, balancing sensual self-entrancement and partner interaction arousal focus, PM relaxation, and cognitive and behavioral arousal pacing.

- Ejaculatory control requires you to identify the point of ejaculatory inevitability and maintain awareness at high levels of arousal.

- Ejaculatory control during partner sex, especially intercourse, is complex and challenging.

- Only one in four women have the same response pattern as men (a single orgasm during intercourse). The goal of ejaculatory control is not to guarantee that your partner has an orgasm during intercourse. The goal is to increase pleasure and eroticism for both of you.

- Three of the most effective behavioral tools are PM relaxation, the stop-start technique, and the intercourse acclimation technique.

- Learning ejaculatory control is a gradual process requiring practice and feedback. If your PE is severe, you should not skip any of the steps in chapter 8.

- Relax your PM as much as possible as you initiate intercourse to give your body some margin for ejaculatory control.

- When you begin learning ejaculatory control during intercourse, begin with the woman-on-top position and be sure to allow enough time for acclimation.

- Other intercourse positions are more challenging. Utilize longer, slower thrusting or circular thrusting. Alternate which partner controls the thrusting. Ejaculatory control is most difficult in the man-on-top position with short, rapid thrusting.

- Sensations of orgasm begin at the point of ejaculatory inevitability. Once you reach the point of inevitability, there's no turning back. Whether you arrive there prematurely or voluntarily, enjoy the feelings and sensations and do not be upset or angry. Beating up on yourself does not facilitate ejaculatory control.

- Your partner's emotional and sexual feelings are very important. Her role is an intimate, involved partner. You can pleasure her to arousal and orgasm with manual, oral, rubbing, or vibrator stimulation. Most women prefer this before ejaculation, but some prefer after. Sex does not end when you ejaculate.

- Remember that you can use medication as an additional resource, especially if you have neurologic system PE (your quick ejaculatory response is hardwired). You can practice ejaculatory control exercises while taking medication and then gradually eliminate medication (be sure to talk with your doctor).

- Sexuality is about giving and receiving pleasure, not performing perfectly. Enjoy and share the entire sexual experience: intimacy, pleasure, eroticism, arousal, intercourse, and afterplay.

Jonathan and Angela's Story

For most of the eight years they had been together (the last six as a married couple), Jonathan had a severe, chronic PE pattern. The sexual problem did not affect Angela's feelings of love for Jonathan or her commitment to the marriage, but it did have a negative impact on their sexual relationship. Angela began to have trouble with sexual desire, arousal, and orgasm.

Jonathan and Angela had a complementary couple style that fit them well in most ways, but sexuality did not play the 15 to 20 percent energizing role. For Angela, sexuality was a disappointment but not a major factor in her life. Their four-year-old son and two-year-old daughter kept them busy; that was Angela's rationale for why they were sexual only two to three times a month. If she asked, Jonathan would manually stimulate her before moving to intercourse, and usually Angela would be orgasmic. However, over time and because of the children, Angela began to settle for quick intercourse and became reluctant to ask for the time and stimulation to meet her sexual needs.

Jonathan did not like to think about the PE problem. He alternated between blaming himself and blaming Angela. Jonathan especially blamed Angela for the infrequency of sex. He wistfully recalled the first eight months of their relationship, when they had sex each time they were together and neither Jonathan nor Angela worried about PE.

It was not until they were engaged that Angela tactfully told Jonathan that she would enjoy sex more if it was slower and more loving. Jonathan wanted to please Angela, but was not clear about what she meant. He did spend more time on kissing and caressing, but as soon as Angela's underwear was off, Jonathan focused on manually stimulating her to orgasm, which he found very arousing. As soon as she was orgasmic he would enter her, and after a few rapid, exciting strokes he would ejaculate. Jonathan felt good about their sexual life; his only complaint was frequency. He assumed she was pleased because she was easily orgasmic with manual stimulation and did not say anything to the contrary.

During and after their first pregnancy (which was wanted and planned), there was a significant decrease in sexual frequency. The second pregnancy was unplanned, but their daughter was very much wanted. Two young children and sleep deprivation wiped out Angela's sexual receptivity and responsivity, but not Jonathan's. They fell into a push-pull power struggle over frequency of intercourse.

After a particularly rushed intercourse, Jonathan asked whether she would like to make love again and offered to stimulate her to orgasm first. Angela felt put upon, and told him so. Jonathan responded in what he thought was a joking manner about mothers not being very sexy. Angela found this objectionable and told him to stop being so self-centered, that he should be glad she was willing to put up with his PE. Jonathan and Angela had fallen into the trap of arguing about sex while naked and vulnerable, right after a sexual encounter—always a bad idea.

Angela wanted to enhance intimacy and pleasuring in the marriage, while Jonathan wanted to increase the frequency of sexual intercourse. These are not incompatible goals, but Angela and Jonathan needed to communicate and work together to improve their sexual relationship.

A crucial step was to determine what type of PE Jonathan had. Together, they completed the PE diagnostic process in chapter 4. Angela encouraged Jonathan to seek help, realizing that his PE was lifelong, occurred in all situations, and was neurologically based. Angela accompanied Jonathan to his appointment with the internist, who agreed that he was suffering from the neurological system type of PE. It was Angela who encouraged a full treatment plan: taking medication, learning psychosexual skills, and increasing empathy and intimacy. Jonathan had been so caught up in embarrassment about having PE that he found it hard to have frank talks about PE and what it meant to Angela and to the relationship.

The internist asked if they wanted a referral to a psychologist or a sex therapist, but they decided to work together to try methods such as those in this book first. Angela said she was open to couple sex therapy if there was not significant improvement after six months. Jonathan was motivated to address PE as a couple, partly because he was anxious about sex therapy. (Typically, men are very willing to attend sex therapy if there is a female dysfunction, but much more hesitant if there is a male dysfunction.)

With Jonathan more aware and motivated, Angela playing an active role in improving psychosexual skills, the use of Zoloft, and increased empathy and cooperation, they saw gradual but quite significant improvement in ejaculatory control and much improvement in sexual frequency and satisfaction. What made the most difference for Jonathan was using pelvic muscle exercises, learning to enjoy slow, sensual stimulation, and utilizing circular thrusting during intercourse. What made the most difference for Angela was increasing nongenital and genital pleasuring, using multiple stimulation during intercourse, and developing enjoyable afterplay scenarios.

The issue that now concerned Jonathan and Angela was how to maintain and generalize their sexual gains and ensure that they did not relapse. Jonathan's biggest question was whether he needed to continue taking medication or could wean himself from it. Angela wanted assurance that even when they no longer had to schedule time to do sexual exercises, they would still make time for each other and nurture their intimate bond. Jonathan made an appointment with his internist, who helped him develop a schedule to slowly reduce medication. Angela told Jonathan that she valued sensual, playful touch as well as erotic touch and intercourse.

The relapse prevention strategy that mattered most to Angela was setting aside couple time every six to eight weeks when there was a specific ban on intercourse. This allowed them to experiment with both sensual and erotic scenarios to maintain a sense of sexual adventure and realize that not all sexual touch had to result in intercourse. The relapse prevention strategy that mattered most to Jonathan was purposefully enjoying the sensations at the plateau phase rather than quickly moving to intercourse, as well as using a variety of intercourse positions and types and rhythms of thrusting. The hardest thing for Jonathan was accepting that it was okay to enjoy the feelings of orgasm when he ejaculated before he would have chosen to. Jonathan accepted that a pleasure orientation was healthier than a performance orientation. When Jonathan did experience a rapid ejaculation lapse, he did not go away but instead held and pleasured Angela. To ensure that he did not become self-conscious about the early ejaculation, they would try to have another sexual encounter in the next one to three days. Jonathan enjoyed spending more time in the pleasuring, intercourse, and afterplay phases.

Even though they had two careers, two growing children, and a busy life, Jonathan and Angela set aside time to be an intimate sexual couple. Sexual intercourse and ejaculatory control were a critical part of their couple sexual style. In addition, they valued and enjoyed a broad-based, flexible relationship that included emotional intimacy, affectionate and sensual touch, playful touching both in and out of the bedroom, enjoying a variety of pleasuring and erotic scenarios, and basking in afterplay. Jonathan and Angela's new couple style valued both marital intimacy and erotic sexuality.

Relapse Prevention Strategies

The best overall relapse prevention strategy is for both you and your partner to commit to devoting the time and energy it takes to maintain a high-quality intimate relationship. This includes maintaining a regular rhythm of affectionate, sensual, playful, and erotic sexual connection—whether three times a week or once every ten days—rather than regressing to the intercourse-or-nothing approach to touching. But healthy sexuality is much more than frequency. A vital sexuality involves attending to physical health and healthy habits (including not smoking, good eating habits, regular exercise, a healthy sleep pattern, and moderate drinking or no drinking). You want to have a good relationship with a primary care physician to ensure that an illness or medication side effect does not interfere with your sexual functioning. You need to be committed to enhancing your personal well-being and the well-being of your partner.

There are ten specific relapse prevention strategies for you to consider.

Strategy One: Hold Couple Meetings

Having regular times (for example, every month) to discuss your intimate relationship is crucial to maintaining a vital relationship. One advantage of working as an intimate team in learning ejaculatory control or being in couple therapy is that you regularly engage in serious communication about your relationship. You want to continue to devote the time and energy to nurture and enhance your intimate relationship. It's important to show your partner your desire to maintain your intimate bond.

Strategy Two: Have a Formal Follow-Up Meeting

Planning a six-month follow-up (by yourselves or with a therapist) will help you remain committed and accountable to good-quality, enjoyable sex and prevent relapse by ensuring that you do not slip back into unhealthy sexual attitudes, behaviors, or feelings. The biggest trap is to treat PE and intimacy with benign neglect. If you don't pay attention, sex will regress to marginal quality and become infrequent.

Strategy Three: Have Pleasuring Sessions

Setting aside time for a pleasuring session (with a prohibition on orgasm) reinforces communication, sensuality, and playfulness. This allows you to enjoy sensuality and experiment with new things: an alternative pleasuring position, body lotion, a new setting or milieu. This helps keep you focused on pleasure and flexibility. Maintaining pleasuring and sensuality combats relapse not just for PE but for other sexual problems as well.

Strategy Four: Calmly Accept Your Lapses as Simple Tests

In any change process, when you begin to achieve reasonable success, you will be tested. This is normal. When your new skills are challenged and you do a good-enough job of handling the test, you will be able to relax, settle in, and feel calmly confident. You will realize that your progress is for real, not a fluke. Your success will become believable. You have learned the skills of sexual cooperation and intimacy.

As a couple, you will likely be tested a minimum of two times. The usual test is a lapse, an experience of PE as severe as it ever was. You will have automatic thoughts of self-doubt: "The treatment approach didn't work!" "We're back where we started from." "Failure!" "We're going to return to the hurt, anger, and frustration." These are normal thoughts, and you actually need to go back to the old experience several times in order to reaffirm for yourselves that these fears are not accurate.

When you are tested, what is important is that you pass the challenge together. You do this by handling the rapid ejaculation with the understanding and physical, emotional, and relationship skills you have learned throughout this book. In other words, while you may ejaculate fast, do not allow yourselves to relapse to handling it in the old dysfunctional way. Rather, accept the quickness, adapt your lovemaking, continue to pleasure and touch, and stay connected. Let it only be an "oops!" event. Afterward, calmly discuss whether you think the quick ejaculation was simply a random event or whether there are some adjustments you will want to make together for the next times you make love. These might include taking more time to relax your bodies, making love more slowly, attending more to relaxing your PM before you initiate intercourse, allowing more time for vaginal acclimation, or using circular intercourse motions. You can smile and shrug off the experience and make a date in the next one to three days when you have the time and energy for a sensuous, slower lovemaking experience.

The better you pass this test, the more assured your success will be. If you don't handle the testing well, it will take more practice at passing more tests to confirm your success. That is why it helps if you consciously anticipate the tests together so that you are not taken off guard.

Strategy Five: Remember to Focus on Reasonable Expectations

We hope that by now you've let go of your ideas about movie-quality sex and erections that last for hours. If sexuality is to remain positive and nurture your intimate bond, you need to keep your expectations reasonable and accept flexibility and variability. Adopt a broad-based approach to touching and eroticism. Remember there are multiple purposes for sex. Allow sexuality to meet a variety of individual and couple needs. Sometimes sex is a tension reducer, sometimes a way to share closeness; other times a short, passionate encounter, a way to heal an argument, a bridge to reduce emotional distance. It is a reality that sex is often better for one partner than the other.

Strategy Six: Schedule Intimate Couple Time

The importance of setting aside quality couple time, especially intimacy dates or weekends without the kids, cannot be emphasized enough. Nurture your relationship intimacy. For couples with children, it is especially important to set aside couple time, whether a night out each week or a weekend away without the children at least once a year. Couples often report better sex on vacation, validating the importance of getting away even for an hour or two. Couple time can include going for a walk, having a sexual date, going to dinner, or having an intimate talk.

Strategy Seven: Let Your Couple Sexual Style Develop over Time

There is not one right way to be sexual. Each couple develops their unique style of initiation, pleasuring, erotic scenarios and techniques, intercourse, and afterplay. The more flexible your couple sexual style and the more you accept the multiple functions of touching and sexuality, the greater your resistance to relapse. Develop a comfortable, functional, satisfying sexual style that meets both of your needs and energizes your relationship.

Strategy Eight: Remember That Good-Enough Sex Ranges from Disappointing to Great

Be prepared to cope with disappointing or negative sexual experiences. The single most important technique in relapse prevention is the ability to accept and not overreact to experiences that are mediocre, unsatisfying, or dysfunctional. Any couple can get along if everything goes well. The challenge is to accept disappointing or dysfunctional experiences without panicking or blaming. Rapid ejaculation, inhibited sexual desire, losing an erection, female non-orgasmic response, a miscommunication about a sexual date: these happen to all couples. Intimate couples accept occasional mediocre or disappointing experiences and take pride in having a resilient sexual style.

Strategy Nine: Saturate Each Other with Multidimensional Touch

Intimacy includes sexuality, but is much more than sexual intercourse. You need a variety of intimate and erotic ways to connect, reconnect, and maintain connection. These include affectionate touch, holding, nongenital pleasuring, playful touch, erotic stimulation, and intercourse. This gives you lots of tools to build bridges to sexual desire. The more ways you have to maintain intimate and sexual connection, the better you can avoid relapse.

Strategy Ten: Keep Expanding Your Sexual Repertoire

The importance of maintaining an erotic relationship and having a variety of sexual alternatives and scenarios cannot be overemphasized. A flexible sexual repertoire is a major antidote to relapse. Sexuality that meets a range of needs, feelings, and situations will serve you well in maintaining ejaculatory control and supporting your sexual and emotional gains. Couples who express intimacy through massage, holding hands, bathing together, enjoying playful touch, engaging in semiclothed cuddling, and enjoying nude sensual touch have a flexible repertoire. Couples who are open to "quickies," prolonged and varied erotic scenarios, various intercourse positions, multiple stimulation during intercourse, and planned as well as spontaneous sexual encounters have a robust sexual relationship.

Choose Your Relapse Prevention Strategies

Now that we have reviewed the ten relapse prevention strategies, your task is to work with your partner to choose two to four that are personally relevant, and then decide how to implement these strategies as part of your individualized relapse prevention plan.

In movies and novels, once the problem is resolved, you expect to live happily ever after. In reality, your relationship and sexuality require attention. We advocate an active relapse prevention program, and if sexuality gets off track, a problem-solving approach. Couples need to be able to deal with rapid ejaculation and other sexual difficulties when they occur, but relapse prevention is easier and more effective. Why waste psychological energy dealing with a crisis when you can more efficiently and happily prevent the problem?

Realistic expectations are a key ingredient in sexual satisfaction. You can accept occasional mediocre, disappointing, or failed sexual experiences. The more broadly based your sexual relationship, with emphasis on sharing desire, pleasure, eroticism, intercourse, and orgasm, the greater the likelihood you will maintain your gains and prevent relapse.

You have come too far to relapse to PE and sexual performance pressure. Confronting PE was a team effort. Maintaining and generalizing intimacy, sexual pleasure, and ejaculatory control is likewise a team process. When people regress to PE, it is usually a result of benign neglect. It is easy to procrastinate, be diverted by other things, fall into old habits, and let intimacy and sexuality slip down your list of priorities. Sexuality should not be the top priority in your relationship, but it should be a positive, integral component. You want to reinforce the positive feedback cycle of anticipation, pleasure, and a regular rhythm of sexual intercourse. Value intimacy, pleasure, and eroticism for yourself and for the relationship. Have great sex together!

Choosing an Individual, Couple, or Sex Therapist

This is a self-help book, but it is not a do-it-yourself therapy book. Men and couples are often reluctant to consult a therapist, feeling that to do so is a sign of craziness, a confession of inadequacy, or an admission that your life and relationship are in dire straits. In reality, seeking professional help is a sign of psychological wisdom and strength. Entering individual, couple, or sex therapy means you realize there is a problem and you have made a commitment to resolve the issues and promote individual and couple growth.

The mental health field can be confusing. Couple and sex therapy are clinical subspecialties. They are offered by several groups of professionals including psychologists, social workers, marriage therapists, psychiatrists, and pastoral counselors. The professional background of the practitioner is less important than his or her competence in dealing with your PE and other specific problems.

Many people have health insurance that provides coverage for mental health, and thus can afford the services of a private practitioner. Those who do not have either the financial resources or insurance could consider a city or county mental health clinic, a university or medical school outpatient mental health clinic, or a family services center. Some clinics have a sliding fee scale (the fee is based on your ability to pay).

When choosing a therapist, be assertive in asking about credentials and areas of expertise. Ask the clinician what will be the focus of the therapy, how long therapy can be expected to last, and whether the emphasis is specifically on sexual problems or more generally on individual, communication, or relationship issues. Be especially diligent in asking about credentials such as university degrees and licensing. Be wary of people who call themselves personal counselors, marriage counselors, or sex counselors. There are poorly qualified people—and some outright quacks—in any field.

One of the best ways to obtain a referral is to call a local professional organization such as a psychological association, marriage and family therapy association, mental health association, or mental health clinic. You can ask for a referral from a family physician, clergy or rabbi, or trusted friend. If you live near a university or medical school, call to find out what mental and sexual health services may be available.

For a sex therapy referral, contact the American Association of Sex Educators, Counselors, and Therapists through the Internet at www.aasect.org or write or call for a list of certified sex therapists in your area: P.O. Box 5488, Richmond, VA 23220; (804) 644-3288. Another resource is the Society for Sex Therapy and Research (SSTAR) at www.sstarnet.org.

For a marital therapist, check the Web sites for the American Association of Marriage and Family Therapy at www.therapistlocator.net or the Association for the Advancement of Behavioral Therapy (AABT) at www.aabt.com.

Feel free to talk with two or three therapists before deciding on one with whom to work. Be aware of your level of comfort with the therapist, degree of rapport, whether the therapist has special skill working with couples, and whether the therapist's assessment of the problem and approach to treatment makes sense to you.

Once you begin, give therapy a chance to be helpful. There are few miracle cures. Change requires commitment and is a gradual and often difficult process. Although some people benefit from short-term therapy (fewer than ten sessions), most find the therapeutic process requires four months to a year or longer. The role of the therapist is that of a consultant rather than a decision maker. Therapy requires effort, both in the session and at home. Therapy helps to change attitudes, feelings, and behavior. Although it takes courage to seek professional help, therapy can be a tremendous help in evaluating and changing individual, relational, and sexual problems.

Resources

Suggested Reading on Male Sexuality

Joannides, Paul. 1999. *The Guide to Getting It On.* West Hollywood, Calif.: The Goofy Foot Press.

McCarthy, Barry, and Emily McCarthy. 1998. *Male Sexual Awareness.* New York: Carroll and Graf.

Milsten, Richard, and Julian Slowinski. 1999. *The Sexual Male: Problems and Solutions.* New York: W. W. Norton & Company.

Zilbergeld, Bernie. 1999. *The New Male Sexuality.* New York: Bantam Books.

Suggested Reading on Female Sexuality

Ellison, Carol. 2001. *Women's Sexualities.* Oakland, Calif.: New Harbinger Publications.

Foley, Sallie, Sally Kope, and Dennis Sugrue. 2002. *Sex Matters for Women: A Complete Guide to Taking Care of Your Sexual Self.* New York: Guilford Publications.

Goodwin, Aurelie, and Marc Agronin. 1997. *A Woman's Guide to Overcoming Sexual Fear and Pain.* Oakland, Calif.: New Harbinger Publications.

Heiman, Julian, and Joseph LoPiccolo. 1988. *Becoming Orgasmic: Women's Guide to Sexual Fulfillment.* New York: Prentice-Hall.

Leiblum, Sandra, and Judith Sachs. 2002. *Getting the Sex You Want: A Woman's Guide to Becoming Proud, Passionate, and Pleased in Bed.* New York: Crown Publishers (Random House).

Suggested Reading on Couple Sexuality

Holstein, Lana. 2002. *How to Have Magnificent Sex: The Seven Dimensions of a Vital Sexual Connection.* New York: Harmony Books (Random House).

McCarthy, Barry, and Emily McCarthy. 1998. *Couple Sexual Awareness.* New York: Carroll and Graf.

————. 2002. *Sexual Awareness.* New York: Carroll and Graf.

Schnarch, David. 2002. *Passionate marriage: Sex, love, and intimacy in emotionally committed relationships.* New York: Norton.

Other Notable Sexuality Readings

Butler, Robert, and Myrna Lewis. 2002. *The New Love and Sex after Sixty.* New York: Ballantine.

Maltz, Wendy. 2001. *The Sexual Healing Journey.* New York: Harper-Collins.

McCarthy, Barry, and Emily McCarthy. 2003. *Rekindling Desire.* New York: Brunner/Routledge.

Michael, Robert, John Gagnon, Edward Laumann, and Gina Kolata. 1994. *Sex in America: A Definitive Survey.* New York: Little, Brown and Company.

Suggested Reading on Relationship Satisfaction

Chapman, Gary. 1995. *The Five Love Languages: How to Express Heartfelt Commitment to Your Mate.* Chicago: Northfield Publishing.

Doherty, William. 2001. *Take Back Your Marriage.* New York: Guilford Press.

Gottman, John. 1999. *The Seven Principles for Making Marriage Work.* New York: Crown Publishing.

Markman, Howard, Scott Stanley, and Susan L. Blumberg. 2001. *Fighting for Your Marriage: Positive Steps for Preventing Divorce and Preserving a Lasting Love.* San Francisco: Jossey-Bass Publishers.

Videotapes: Ejaculatory Control Techniques

Desjardins, Jean-Yves, and Nicole Audette. 1997. *The Lover's Guide to Ejaculatory Control.* 55 min.
Pacific Media Entertainment, P.O. Box 4326, Chatsworth, CA 91311.
Fax (818) 341-3562.
www.pacificmediaent.com.

Polonsky, Derek, and Marian Dunn. 1991. *You Can Last Longer.* Vol. 8, Better Sex Videos Series. 38 min.
Distributor: Sinclair Intimacy Institute, P.O. Box 8865, Chapel Hill, NC 27515.
(800) 955-0888. Fax (800) 794-3318.
www.bettersex.com.

Videotapes: Sexual Enrichment

The Couples Intimacy Guide to Great Sex over 40, vols. 1 and 2. 1995. 60 min.
Sinclair Institute, P.O. Box 8865, Chapel Hill, NC 27515.
(800) 955-0888. Fax (800) 794-3318.
www.bettersex.com.

Holstein, Lana. 2001. *Magnificent Lovemaking.* 79 min.
Canyon Ranch Bookstore, Tucson, AZ. 85750
(520) 749-9000, extension 4380.

Perry, Michael, and Goedele Liekens. 1991. *Sex: A Lifelong Pleasure* series.
Sinclair Intimacy Institute, P.O. Box 8865, Chapel Hill, NC 27515.
(800) 955-0888. Fax (800) 794-3318.
www.bettersex.com.

Sommers, Frank. *The Great Sex Video Series.* Distributor: Pathway Productions, Inc., 360 Bloor Street West, Suite 407A, Toronto M5S 1X1, Canada.
(416) 922-4506. Fax (416) 922-7512.
E-mail: how2video@ aol.com.

Stubbs, Kenneth Ray. 1994. *Erotic Massage.* 58 min.
Secret Garden, P.O. Box 67, Larkspur, CA 94977.

Professional Associations

American Association of Sex Educators, Counselors, and Therapists (AASECT): P.O. Box 54388, Richmond, VA 23220-0488.
www.aasect.org.
(804) 644-3288

Association for the Advancement of Behavioral Therapy (AABT): 305 Seventh Avenue, New York, NY 10001-6008.
(212) 647-1890.
www.aabt.org.

Sex Information and Education Council of the United States (SIECUS): 130 West 42nd Street, Suite 350, New York, NY 10036.
(212) 819-7990. Fax (212) 819-9776.
www.seicus.org.

Society for Scientific Study of Sexuality (SSSS): David Fleming, Executive Director. P.O. Box 416, Allentown, PA 18105-0416.
(610) 530-2483.
www.sexscience.org.

Society for Sex Therapy and Research (SSTAR): www.sstarnet.org.

Sex "Toys," Books, and Videos

Good Vibrations Mail Order: 938 Howard Sreet, Suite 101, San Francisco, CA 94110.
(800) 289-8423. Fax (415) 974-8990.
www.goodvibes.com.

References

Assalian, P. 1988. Clomipramine in the treatment of premature ejaculation. *Journal of Sex Research* 4:213–215.

Basson, R. 2001. Using a different model for female sexual response to address women's problematic low sexual desire. *Journal of Sex and Marital Therapy* 27:395–403.

Bixler, R. H. 1986. Of apes and men (including females!). *Journal of Sex Research* 20:109–12.

Epstein, N., and D. Baucom. 2002. *Enhanced Cognitive Behavioral Therapy for Couples: A Contextual Approach.* Washington, D.C.: American Psychological Association.

Foley, S., S. Kope, and D. Sugrue. 2002. *Sex Matters for Women: A Complete Guide to Taking Care of Your Sexual Self.* New York: Guilford Publications.

Frank, E., C. Anderson, and D. Rubenstein. 1978. Frequency of sexual dysfunction in "normal" couples. *New England Journal of Medicine* 229(3): 111–15.

Hong, K. 1984. Survival of the fastest: On the origin of premature ejaculation. *Journal of Sex Research* 20:109–12.

Kaplan, H. S. 1974. *The New Sex Therapy.* New York: Brunner/Mazel.

Kinsey, A. C., B. W. Pomeroy, and C. E. Martin. 1948. *Sexual Behavior in the Human Male.* Philadelphia: W. B. Saunders.

La Pera, G., and A. Nicastro. 1996. A new treatment for premature ejaculation: The rehabilitation of the pelvic floor. *Journal of Sex and Marital Therapy* 22:22–26.

Laumann, E., A. Paik, and R. Rosen. 1999. Sexual dysfunction in the United States: Prevalence and predictors. *Journal of the American Medical Association* 261:537–44.

Leiblum, S., and R. Rosen, eds. 1989. *Principles and Practice of Sex Therapy: Update for the 1990s.* New York: Guilford Publications.

Loudon, J. B. 1988. Potential confusion between erectile dysfunction and premature ejaculation: An evaluation of men presenting with erectile difficulty at a sex therapy clinic. *Journal of Sex and Marital Therapy* 13(4):397–401.

Masters, W. H., and V. E. Johnson. 1966. *Human Sexual Response.* Boston: Little, Brown and Company.

———. 1970. *Human Sexual Inadequacy.* Boston: Little, Brown and Company.

Michael, R., J. Gagnon, E. Laumann, and G. Kolata. 1994. *Sex in America: A Definitive Survey.* New York: Little, Brown and Company.

Mosher, D. L. 1980. Three psychological dimensions of depth of involvement in human sexual response. *Journal of Sex Research* 16(1):1–42.

Rowland, D. L. 1999. Issues in the laboratory study of human sexual response: A synthesis for the nontechnical sexologist. *Journal of Sex Research* 36:1–13.

Schapiro, B. 1943. Premature ejaculation: A review of 1130 cases. *Journal of Urology* 50:374–79.

Semans, J. H. 1956. Premature ejaculation: A new approach. *South Medical Journal* 49:353–58.

Tullii, R. E., C. H. Guillaux, R. Vaccari, and R. Ferreira. 1994. Premature ejaculation selective neurotomy: A new therapeutic technique. Basis, indication, and results. *International Journal of Impotence Research* 6 Suppl. 1P:109-104-103.

Waldinger, M. 1998. Familial occurrence of primary premature ejaculation. *Psychiatric Genetics* 8:37–40.

Wise, M., and J. Watson. 2002. A new treatment for premature ejaculation: Case series for a desensitizing band. *Sexual and Relationship Therapy* 15(4):345–50.

We Want Your Candid Feedback:

We are very interested in your response to our book and welcome your feedback!

For example:

- Why did you buy our book?

- What has been helpful to you?

- What about our approach do you like?

- What do you wish we had addressed more fully?

Please send an email or letter with your comments, requests, or ideas to:

CopingWithPE@aol.com

Or:

Michael E. Metz, Ph.D.
Meta Associates
Baker Court, Suite 440,
821 Raymond Avenue
St. Paul, Minnesota 55114
MMetzMpls@aol.com

Barry W. McCarthy, Ph.D.
Washington Psychological Center
4201 Connecticut Avenue, N.W.
Suite 602
Washington, DC 20008
McCarthy160@comcast.net

We Welcome Your Requests:

We also welcome requests to present workshops, training sessions, and lectures about PE, sexual health, marital and sexual wellness, and couple conflict.

Thank you very much. Michael Metz and Barry McCarthy

Michael Metz, Ph.D., works in the Twin Cities of Minneapolis–St. Paul, Minnesota and is the country's leading sexologist in the area of PE. He is a major spokesperson for a comprehensive, integrated bio-psychosocial approach to addressing and resolving sexual problems. After twelve years on the faculty of the University of Minnesota Medical School, he currently works in private practice with Meta Associates as a psychologist, marital therapist, and sex therapist treating individuals and couples, and is affiliated with the University of Minnesota's Department of Family Social Science. He has published more than forty-five professional articles and conducted numerous workshops and talks on marital and sex therapy. He is the author of the *Styles of Conflict Inventory (SCI)*, a clinical assessment instrument to evaluate the conflict patterns in relationships.

Barry McCarthy, Ph.D., is a clinical psychologist, with a subspecialty in marriage and sex therapy, practicing at the Washington Psychological Center in Washington, DC. He is professor of psychology at American University where he teaches an undergraduate human sexual behavior course. Barry, with his wife Emily, has written seven well-respected books, the most recent being *Getting It Right the First Time, Sexual Awareness*, and *Rekindling Desire*. In addition, Barry has published over fifty-five professional articles, fourteen book chapters, and presented over one hundred and ten workshops nationally and internationally.

Some Other
New Harbinger Titles

A Cancer Patient's Guide to Overcoming Depression and Anxiety,
    Item 5044 $19.95
The Diabetes Lifestyle Book, Item 5167 $16.95
Solid to the Core, Item 4305 $14.95
Staying Focused in the Age of Distraction, Item 433X $16.95
Living Beyond Your Pain, Item 4097 $19.95
Fibromyalgia & Chronic Fatigue Syndrome, Item 4593 $14.95
Your Miraculous Back, Item 4526 $18.95
TriEnergetics, Item 4453 $15.95
Emotional Fitness for Couples, Item 4399 $14.95
The MS Workbook, Item 3902 $19.95
Depression & Your Thyroid, Item 4062 $15.95
The Eating Wisely for Hormonal Balance Journal, Item 3945 $15.95
Healing Adult Acne, Item 4151 $15.95
The Memory Doctor, Item 3708 $11.95
The Emotional Wellness Way to Cardiac Health, Item 3740 $16.95
The Cyclothymia Workbook, Item 383X $18.95
The Matrix Repatterning Program for Pain Relief, Item 3910 $18.95
Transforming Stress, Item 397X $10.95
Eating Mindfully, Item 3503 $13.95
Living with RSDS, Item 3554 $16.95
The Ten Hidden Barriers to Weight Loss, Item 3244 $11.95
The Sjogren's Syndrome Survival Guide, Item 3562 $15.95
Stop Feeling Tired, Item 3139 $14.95
Responsible Drinking, Item 2949 $19.95
The Mitral Valve Prolapse/Dysautonomia Survival Guide, Item 3031 $14.95
The Vulvodynia Survival Guide, Item 2914 $16.95
The Multifidus Back Pain Solution, Item 2787 $12.95

Call **toll free, 1-800-748-6273,** or log on to our online bookstore at **www.newharbinger.com** to order. Have your Visa or Mastercard number ready. Or send a check for the titles you want to New Harbinger Publications, Inc., 5674 Shattuck Ave., Oakland, CA 94609. Include $4.50 for the first book and 75¢ for each additional book, to cover shipping and handling. (California residents please include appropriate sales tax.) Allow two to five weeks for delivery.

Prices subject to change without notice.